Neuroscience at a Glance

Neuroscience at a Glance

ROGER A. BARKER

BA, MBBS, MRCP, PhD
Cambridge Centre for Brain Repair and Department of Neurology
University of Cambridge
Robinson Way
Cambridge

STEPHEN BARASI

BSc, PhD
School of Bioscience
Cardiff University
Museum Avenue
Cardiff

and Neuropharmacology by

MICHAEL J. NEAL

DSc, PhD, MA, BPharm
Professor and Chairman of the
Division of Pharmacology and Toxicology
United Medical and Dental Schools of Guy's and St Thomas's Hospitals (UMDS)
Department of Pharmacology
St Thomas's Hospital, London

SECOND EDITION

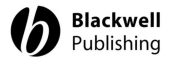

Blackwell
Publishing

© 1999, 2003 by Blackwell Publishing Ltd
Blackwell Publishing, Inc., 350 Main Street, Malden, Massachusetts 02148-5020, USA
Blackwell Publishing Ltd, 9600 Garsington Road, Oxford OX4 2DQ, UK
Blackwell Publishing Asia Pty Ltd, 550 Swanston Street, Carlton South, Victoria 3053, Australia

First published 1999
Reprinted 2000 (twice), 2001, 2003
Second edition 2003
Reprinted 2004

Library of Congress Cataloging-in-Publication Data

Barker, Roger A., 1961–
    Neuroscience at a glance/Roger A. Barker, Stephen Barasi;
    and Neuropharmacology by Michael J. Neal. — 2nd ed.
        p. ; cm.
    Includes index.
    ISBN 1-4051-1124-0
    1 Neurosciences.
    [DNLM: 1 Nervous System Physiology. 2 Nervous System Diseases.
    WL 102 B2557n 2003] I Barasi, Stephen. II Neal, M. J. III Title.

    RC341.B326 2003
    612.8 — dc21
                                                                2003004943

ISBN 1-4051-1124-0

A catalogue record for this title is available from the British Library

Set in 9/11.5 Times by SNP Best-set Typesetter Ltd., Hong Kong
Printed and bound in the United Kingdom by Ashford Colour Press, Gosport

Commissioning Editor: Fiona Goodgame
Managing Editor: Geraldine Jeffers
Production Editor: Fiona Pattison
Production Controller: Kate Charman

For further information on Blackwell Publishing, visit our website:
http://www.blackwellpublishing.com

Contents

Introduction 7
List of abbreviations 8

Part 1 The anatomical and functional organization of the nervous system

1   The organization of the nervous system 10
2   The development of the nervous system 12
3   The cells of the nervous system I: Neurones 14
4   The cells of the nervous system II: Neuroglial cells 16
5   Ion channels 18
6   The resting membrane and action potential 20
7   The neuromuscular junction and synapses 22
8   Nerve conduction and synaptic integration 24
9   Neurotransmitters, receptors and their pathways 26
10 Skeletal muscle structure 28
11 Skeletal muscle contraction 30
12 The organization of the spinal cord 32
13 Anatomy of the brainstem 34
14 Cranial nerves 36
15 The organization of the cerebral cortex 38
16 Meninges and cerebrospinal fluid 40
17 Blood supply of the central nervous system 42

Part 2 Sensory systems

18 Sensory systems: an overview 44
19 Sensory transduction 46
20 The somatosensory system 48
21 Pain systems I: Nocioceptors and nocioceptive pathways 50
22 Pain systems II: Pharmacology and management 52
23 The visual system I: The eye and retina 54
24 The visual system II: The visual pathways and subcortical visual areas 56
25 The visual system III: Visual cortical areas 58
26 The auditory system I: The ear and cochlea 60
27 The auditory system II: The auditory pathways and language 62
28 The vestibular system 64
29 Olfaction and taste 66
30 Association cortices: the posterior parietal and prefrontal cortex 68
31 Clinical disorders of the sensory pathways 70

Part 3 Motor systems

32 The organization of the motor systems 72
33 The muscle spindle and lower motorneurone 74
34 Spinal cord motor organization and locomotion 76
35 The cortical motor areas 78
36 Primary motor cortex 80
37 The cerebellum 82
38 The basal ganglia: anatomy and physiology 84
39 Basal ganglia diseases and their treatment 86
40 Eye movements 88
41 Clinical disorders of the motor system 90

Part 4 Autonomic, limbic, brainstem systems and plasticity

42 Autonomic nervous system 92
43 The hypothalamus 94
44 The reticular formation and sleep 96
45 The limbic system, long-term potentiation and memory 98
46 Neural plasticity and neurotrophic factors I: The peripheral nervous system 100
47 Neural plasticity and neurotrophic factors II: The central nervous system 102

Part 5 Disorders of the nervous system

48 Examination of the nervous system 104
49 Investigation of the nervous system 106
50 Neurochemical disorders I: Affective disorders and schizophrenia 108
51 Neurochemical disorders II: Anxiety 110
52 Neurodegenerative disorders 112
53 Neurophysiological disorders: epilepsy 114
54 Neuroimmunological disorders 116
55 Neurogenetic disorders 118

Appendix 1: Major neurotransmitter types 120
Appendix 2a: Ascending sensory pathways in the spinal cord 121
Appendix 2b: Descending motor tracts 121
Appendix 3: Functional and anatomical systems of the cerebellum 122
Index 123

Introduction

Neuroscience at a Glance is designed primarily for undergraduate medical students as a revision text or review of basic neuroscience mechanisms, rather than a comprehensive account of the field of medical neuroscience. The book does not attempt to provide a systematic review of clinical neurology. However, it should also be of use for those in clinical training and practice wanting a review and synopsis of the science behind the clinical practice.

The changing nature of medical training in this country has meant that rather than teaching being discipline based (anatomy, physiology, pharmacology, etc.), the current approach is much more integrated with the focus on the entire system. Students pursuing a problem-based learning course will also benefit from the concise presentation of integrated material.

This book summarizes the rapidly expanding field of neuroscience with reference to clinical disorders, such that the material is set in a clinical context. In general, the later chapters contain more clinical material while the earlier ones contain a section towards the end outlining applied neuroscience. However, learning about the organization of the nervous system purely from clinical disorders is short-sighted as the changing nature of medical neuroscience means that areas with little clinical relevance today may become more of an issue in the future. An example of this is ion channels and the recent burgeoning of a host of channelopathies. For this reason some chapters focus more on scientific mechanisms with less clinical emphasis.

Each chapter presents the bulk of its information in the form of an annotated figure, which is expanded in the accompanying text. It is recommended that the figure is worked through with the text rather than just viewed in isolation. The condensed nature of each chapter means that much of the information has to be given in a didactic fashion, but a list of suggested further reading for each chapter is given on the Blackwell Publishing website, see back cover. Although the text focuses on core material, some additional important detail is also included.

The book has broadly been divided up into sections on the structure and biophysics of the nervous system (Chapters 1–17); the sensory components of the nervous system (Chapters 18–31); the motor components of the nervous system (Chapters 32–41); the autonomic, limbic and brainstem systems underlying wakefulness and sleep along with neural plasticity (Chapters 42–47) and, finally, a section on the approach, investigation and range of clinical disorders of the nervous system (Chapters 48–55). A list of further reading and glossaries of neurological conditions and neuroscientific terms are available free of charge from the Blackwell Publishing website, see the back cover for further details.

Each section builds on the previous ones to some extent, and so reading the introductory chapter may give a greater understanding to later chapters in that section; for example, the somatosensory system chapter may be better read after the chapter on the general organization of sensory systems.

Acknowledgements
Second edition

In this new edition of the book we have updated some of the subjects but the major changes have involved including a little more on the clinical side, given the increasing integration of neuroscience into clinical neurology and vice versa. Therefore there are new chapters on the examination and investigation of the nervous system and summary chapters on motor and sensory disorders at the end of sections 3 and 2, although the clinical emphasis at the end of each chapter is maintained. The chapters have also been slightly re-ordered with the chapters on neural plasticity moving into section 4, following on from the limbic system and long-term potentiation.

This book has evolved out of our teaching of the last few years and the feedback that we have received about the book. We would like to thank Fiona Goodgame and Geraldine Jeffers at Blackwell Publishing, and Alasdair Coles in Cambridge for his patient and inspired reading and suggestions for the new edition.

Roger Barker and Stephen Barasi
Cambridge and Cardiff
November 2002

First edition

The focus and content of *Neuroscience at a Glance* owes a great deal to the numerous groups of students who have wrestled with the difficult and rapidly changing subject of neuroscience. There are a large number of people we would like to thank for their help in the writing of this book; this includes our colleagues at Cambridge and Cardiff who have patiently read through the various drafts of the manuscript and given their honest opinion. In addition, we would especially like to thank Andrew Larner for diligently correcting the wayward ways of our writing and highlighting errors or poorly formulated explanations and Mike Neal for his important sections on neuropharmacology which have provided valuable additional information.

We would also like to thank Mike Stein and Patricia Hardcastle at Blackwell Science for their endless enthusiasm, support and encouragement for this project. Finally, we would like to thank our families for allowing us to spend so much time on this book.

Roger Barker & Stephen Barasi
Cambridge & Cardiff
May 1998

List of abbreviations

5-HIAA	5-hydroxy indole acetic acid
5-HT	5-hydroxytryptamine (serotonin)
A1	primary auditory cortex
ACA	anterior cerebral artery
ACh	acetylcholine
AChE	acetylcholinesterase
AChR	acetylcholine receptor
ACTH	adenocorticotrophic hormone
ADH	antidiuretic hormone (vasopressin)
ADP	adenosine diphosphate
AICA	anterior inferior cerebellar artery
ALS	amyotrophic lateral sclerosis
AMPA-R	α amino-3-hydroxy-5-methyl-4-isoxazole proprionic acid glutamate receptor
ANS	autonomic nervous system
APP	amyloid precursor protein
ATP	adenosine triphosphate
AuD	autosomal dominant
AuR	autosomal recessive
BBB	blood–brain barrier
BM	basilar membrane
BMP	bone morphogenic protein
cAMP	cyclic adenosine monophosphate
CBM	cerebellum
CBP	calcium-binding protein
CCK	cholecystokinin
cf	climbing fibre
cGMP	cyclic guanosine monophosphate
CMCT	central motor conduction time
CMUA	continuous motor unit activity
CNS	central nervous system
COMT	catecholamine-O-methyltransferase
CoST	corticospinal tract
CPG	central pattern generator
CPK	creatine phosphokinase
CSF	cerebrospinal fluid
CT	computerized tomography
CVA	cerebrovascular accident
DA	dopamine
DAG	diacylglycerol
DAT	dementia of the Alzheimer type
dB	decibel
DC	dorsal column
DCN	dorsal column nuclei
DCochN	dorsal cochlear nucleus
DCNN	deep cerebellar nuclei neurone
DMD	Duchenne's muscular dystrophy
DNA	deoxyribonucleic acid
DRG	dorsal root ganglia
DSCT	dorsal spinocerebellar tract
ECG	electrocardiography/electrocardiogram
ECT	electroconvulsive therapy
EEG	electroencephalography/electroencephalogram
EMG	electromyography/electromyogram
enk	enkephalin

EP	evoked potential
epp	end-plate potential
EPSP	excitatory postsynaptic potential
FEF	frontal eye field
fMRI	functional magnetic resonance imaging
FSH	follicle-stimulating hormone
GABA	γ-aminobutyric acid
GABA-R	γ-aminobutyric acid receptor
GAD	glutamic acid decarboxylase
GDNF	glial cell line derived neurotrophic factor
Glut-R	glutamate receptor
GoC	Golgi cell
G_{olf}	G-protein associated with olfactory receptors
GPe	globus pallidus external segment
GPi	globus pallidus internal segment
G-protein	guanosine triphosphate-binding protein
GrC	granule cell
GTO	Golgi tendon organ
GTP	guanosine triphosphate
HLA	histocompatibility locus antigen
HMM	heavy meromyosin
HMSN	hereditary motor sensory neuropathy
HTM	high-threshold mechanoreceptor
Hz	hertz
IC	inferior colliculus
ICA	internal carotid artery
IHC	inner hair cell
IL	intralaminar nuclei of the thalamus
IN	interneurone
IP_3	inositol triphosphate
IPSP	inhibitory postsynaptic potential
JPS	joint position sense
LEMS	Lambert–Eaton myasthenic syndrome
LGMD	limb girdle muscular dystrophy
LGN	lateral geniculate nucleus of the thalamus
LH	luteinizing hormone
LMM	light meromyosin
LMN	lower motorneurone
LTD	long-term depression
LTP	long-term potentiation
MAO	monoamine oxidase
MAO_A	monoamine oxidase type A
MAO_B	monoamine oxidase type B
MAOI	monoamine oxidase inhibitor
MCA	middle cerebral artery
MD	mediodorsal nucleus of the thalamus
mepp	miniature end-plate potential
MGN	medial geniculate nucleus of the thalamus
MHC	major histocompatibility complex
MLF	medial longitudinal fasciculus
MN	motorneurone
MND	motorneurone disease
MRA	magnetic resonance angiography
MRI	magnetic resonance imaging
MRV	magnetic resonance venography

MsI	primary motor cortex	SA	slowly adapting receptor
MUSK	muscle specific kinase	SMA	supplementary motor area
NA	noradrenaline (norepinephrine)	SmI	primary somatosensory cortex
NCS	nerve conduction studies	SmII	secondary somatosensory area
NFT	neurofibrillary tangle	SNAP	soluble NSF attachment protein
NGF	nerve growth factor	SNARE	SNAP receptor
NMDA	N-methyl-D-aspartate	SNc	substantia nigra pars compacta
NMDA-R	N-methyl-D aspartate glutamate receptor	SNP	senile neuritic plaques
NMJ	neuromuscular junction	SNr	substantia nigra pars reticulata
NS	neostriatum	SOC	superior olivary complex
OD	ocular dominance	SP	substance P
OHC	outer hair cell	SPECT	single photon emission computed tomography
PAG	periaqueductal grey matter	SR	sarcoplasmic reticulum
PCA	posterior cerebral artery	SSRI	selective serotonin reuptake inhibitor
PDE	phosphodiesterase	STN	subthalamic nucleus
PET	positron emission tomography	STT	spinothalamic tract
pf	parallel fibre	SVZ	subventricular zone
PGO	pontine–geniculo-occipital	SWS	slow-wave sleep
PICA	posterior inferior cerebellar artery	TENS	transcutaneous nerve stimulation
PMC	premotor cortex	TeST	tectospinal tract
PMN	polymodal nociceptors	TIA	transient ischaemic attack
PMP	peripheral myelin protein	TM	tectorial membrane
PNS	peripheral nervous system	TRH	thyrotrophin-releasing hormone
PPC	posterior parietal cortex	T-tubule	transverse tubule
PPN	pedunculopontine nucleus	UMN	upper motorneurone
PPRF	paramedian pontine reticular formation	V1	primary visual cortex (Brodmann's area 17)
PuC	Purkinje cell	VA–VL	ventroanterior–ventrolateral nuclei of the thalamus
RA	rapidly adapting receptor	VCN	ventral cochlear nucleus
REM	rapid eye movement	VEP	visual evoked potential
ReST	reticulospinal tract	VeST	vestibulospinal tract
RiMLF	rostral interstitial nucleus of the medial longitudinal fasciculus	VOR	vestibulo-ocular reflex
		VP	ventroposterior nucleus of the thalamus
RMS	rostral migratory stream	VPL	ventroposterior nucleus of the thalamus, lateral part
RN	raphe nucleus	VPM	ventroposterior nucleus of the thalamus, medial part
RNA	ribonucleic acid	VPT	vibration perception threshold
RuST	rubrospinal tract	VSCT	ventral spinocerebellar tract

1 The organization of the nervous system

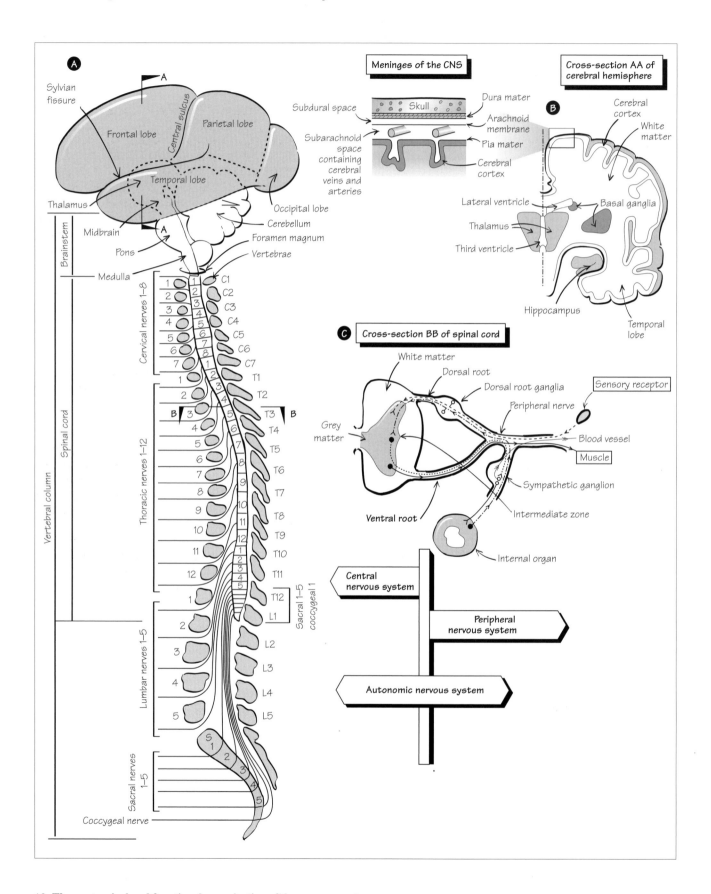

An overview

The nervous system can be divided into three major parts: the **peripheral** (PNS), **central** (CNS) and **autonomic** (ANS) **nervous system**. The PNS is defined as those nerves that lie outside the brain, brainstem or spinal cord, while the CNS embraces those cells that lie within these structures.

Peripheral nervous system

The PNS consists of nerve trunks made up of both afferent fibres or axons conducting sensory information to the spinal cord and brainstem, and efferent fibres transmitting impulses primarily to the muscles. Damage to an individual nerve leads to weakness of the muscles it innervates and sensory loss in the area from which it conveys sensory information. The peripheral nerves occasionally form a dense network or plexus adjacent to the spinal cord (e.g. brachial plexus in the upper limb). The peripheral nerves connect with the spinal cord through foramina between the bones (or **vertebrae**) of the spine (or **vertebral column**), or with the brain through foramina in the skull.

Spinal cord

The **spinal cord** begins at the **foramen magnum**, which is the site in the base of the skull where the lower part of the brainstem (medulla) ends. The spinal cord terminates in the adult at the first lumbar vertebra, and gives rise to 30 pairs (or 31 if the coccygeal nerves are included) of spinal nerves, which exit the spinal cord between the vertebral bones of the spine. The first eight spinal nerves originate from the **cervical spinal cord** with the first pair exiting above the first cervical vertebra and the next 12 spinal nerves originate from the **thoracic or dorsal spinal cord**. The remaining 10 pairs of spinal nerves originate from the lower cord, five from the **lumbar** and five from the **sacral** regions.

The spinal nerves consist of an **anterior or ventral root** that innervates the skeletal muscles, while the **posterior or dorsal root** carries sensation to the spinal cord from the skin that shared a common embryological origin during development with that part of the spinal cord (see Chapter 2). In the case of the dorsal root fibres, they have their cell bodies in the **dorsal root ganglia** which lie just outside the spinal canal.

The spinal cord itself consists of **white matter**, which is that part of it containing the nerve fibres that form the **ascending and descending pathways of the spinal cord**, while the **grey matter** is located in the centre of the spinal cord and contains the cell bodies of the neurones (see Chapter 12).

Brainstem, cranial nerves and cerebellum

The spinal cord gives way to the **brainstem** which lies at the base of the brain and is composed of the **medulla, pons and midbrain** (or mesencephalon) and contains discrete collections of neurones or nuclei for 10 of the 12 cranial nerves (see Chapter 14). The brainstem and the **cerebellum** constitute the structures of the posterior fossa. The cerebellum is connected to the brainstem via three pairs of cerebellar peduncles, and is involved in the coordination of movement (see Chapter 37).

Cerebral hemispheres

The **cerebral hemispheres** are composed of **four major lobes: occipital, parietal, temporal and frontal**. On the medial part of the temporal lobe are a series of structures, including the **hippocampus**, that form the limbic system (see Chapter 45).

The outer layer of the cerebral hemisphere is termed the **cerebral cortex**, and contains neurones that are organized both in horizontal layers and vertical columns (see Chapter 15). The cerebral cortex is interconnected over long distances via pathways that run subcortically. These pathways, together with those that connect the cerebral cortex to the spinal cord, brainstem and nuclei deep within the cerebral hemisphere, constitute **the white matter of the cerebral hemisphere**. These deep nuclei include structures such as the **basal ganglia** (see Chapters 38 and 39) and the **thalamus**.

Meninges

The CNS is enclosed within the skull and vertebral column and separating these structures are a series of membranes known as the **meninges**. The **pia mater** is separated from the delicate **arachnoid membrane** by the subarachnoid space, which in turn is separated from the **dura mater** by the subdural space (see Chapter 16).

Autonomic nervous system

The **ANS** has both a central and peripheral component and is concerned with the innervation of internal and glandular organs (see Chapter 42): it has an important role in the control of the endocrine and homoeostatic systems of the body (see Chapter 43). The peripheral component of the autonomic nervous system is defined in terms of the **enteric, sympathetic and parasympathetic systems** (see Chapter 42).

The efferent fibres of the ANS originate either from the **intermediate zone** (or **lateral column**) of the spinal cord or specific cranial nerve and sacral nuclei and synapse in a **ganglion**, the site of which is different for the sympathetic and parasympathetic systems. The afferent fibres from the organs innervated by the ANS pass via the dorsal root to the spinal cord.

2 The development of the nervous system

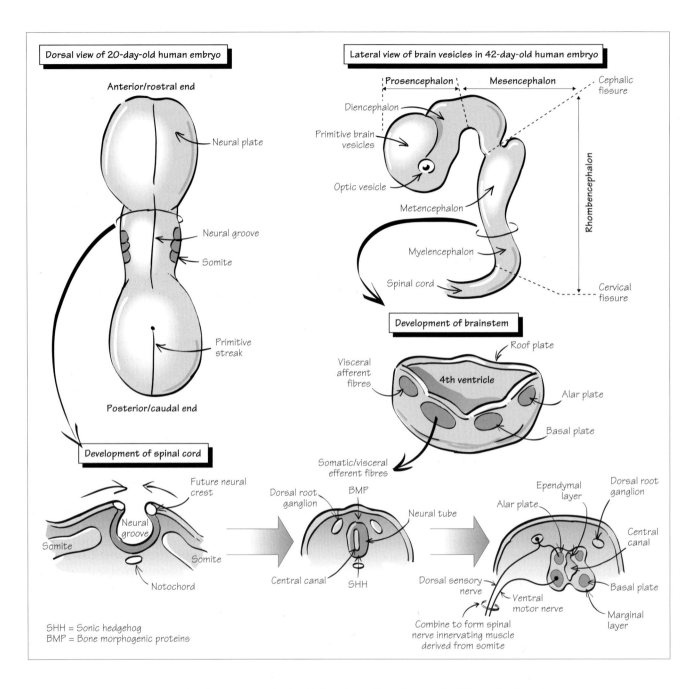

Dorsal view of 20-day-old human embryo

Anterior/rostral end

Neural plate

Neural groove

Somite

Primitive streak

Posterior/caudal end

Development of spinal cord

Future neural crest

Neural groove

Somite

Somite

Notochord

SHH = Sonic hedgehog
BMP = Bone morphogenic proteins

Lateral view of brain vesicles in 42-day-old human embryo

Prosencephalon

Mesencephalon

Cephalic fissure

Diencephalon

Primitive brain vesicles

Optic vesicle

Metencephalon

Myelencephalon

Spinal cord

Rhombencephalon

Cervical fissure

Development of brainstem

Roof plate

Visceral afferent fibres

4th ventricle

Alar plate

Basal plate

Somatic/visceral efferent fibres

Dorsal root ganglion

BMP

Neural tube

Central canal

SHH

Dorsal sensory nerve

Ventral motor nerve

Combine to form spinal nerve innervating muscle derived from somite

Ependymal layer

Dorsal root ganglion

Alar plate

Central canal

Basal plate

Marginal layer

The first signs of nervous system development occur in the third week of gestation, under the influence of secreted factors from the **notochord**, with the formation of a **neural plate** along the dorsal aspect of the embryo. This plate broadens, folds (forming the **neural groove**) and fuses to form the **neural tube** which ultimately gives rise to the brain at its rostral end and the spinal cord caudally. This fusion begins approximately halfway along the neural groove at the level of the fourth somite and continues caudally and rostrally with the closure of the posterior/caudal and anterior/rostral neuropore during the fourth week of gestation. Abnormalities in this process of neuropore closure result in *anencephaly* at the rostral end and certain forms of *spina bifida* at the caudal end (see below).

Development of the spinal cord

The process of neural tube fusion isolates a group of cells termed the **neural crest**. This structure gives rise a range of cells including the **dorsal root ganglia** (DRG) and peripheral components of the ANS. The DRG contain the sensory cell bodies which send their developing axons into the evolving spinal cord and skin. These growing neuronal processes or neurites have an advancing **growth cone** that finds its appropriate target in the periphery and CNS, using a number of cues including cell adhesion molecules and diffusable neurotrophic factors (see Chapter 46).

The neural tube surrounds the neural canal which forms the central canal of the fully developed spinal cord. The tube itself contains the neuroblasts with those adjacent to the canal (**ependymal layer**) dividing and migrating out to the **mantle layer** where they differentiate into neurones and by so doing form the grey matter of the spinal cord (see Chapter 1). The developing processes from the neuroblasts/neurones grow out into the **marginal layer** which therefore ultimately forms the white matter of the spinal cord. The dividing neuroblasts segregate into two discrete populations, the **alar** and **basal plates**, which in turn will form the dorsal and ventral horns of the spinal cord while a small lateral horn of visceral efferent neurones (part of the ANS) develops at their interface in the thoracic and upper lumbar cord (see Chapter 42). This dorsal–ventral patterning relies, at least in part, on secreted factors from the dorsally located notochord (sonic hedgehog) and ventrally on bone morphogenic proteins (BMPs).

Development of the brain

The rostral part of the neural tube enlarges before closure with the formation of three **primary brain vesicles (the prosencephalon, mesencephalon and rhombencephalon)** and two **flexures (cervical and cephalic)**. The primary brain vesicles develop into the cerebral hemispheres, brainstem and cerebellum while the neural canal will ultimately form the ventricular system of the brain (see Chapter 16).

The **prosencephalon** consists of the telencephalon which forms the cerebral hemispheres and part of the basal ganglia while the **diencephalon** forms the thalamus, hypothalamus, posterior pituitary and optic nerve and retina.

The neuroblasts again originate adjacent to the neural canal (the ventricular zone) but in this case they migrate not only locally to form the deep subcortical nuclei of the brain but also out along developing radial glial fibres to form the cerebral cortex (see Chapter 15). This intervening area, which is rich in glial fibres, will ultimately form the white matter of the cerebral hemisphere, with some of the radial glia giving rise to neural precursor cells in the adult brain (see below). The signals involved in the organization of these migrating neurones to and in the cortex are being identified, and defects in these may cause *cortical dysplasia*.

The **mesencephalon** gives rise to the midbrain with the neural canal forming the central aqueduct of Sylvius while the **rhombencephalon** consists of the **metencephalon** that gives rise to the pons and cerebellum and the **myelencephalon** that forms the medulla (see Chapter 13). The brainstem develops in a similar fashion to the spinal cord except the development is in a more mediolateral than anteroposterior direction. Thus, the developing motor nuclei lie medial to the sensory nuclei with a parasympathetic component interposed between the two. This anterolateral expansion therefore explains the organization of the cranial nerve nuclei within the brainstem (see Chapters 13 and 14).

The cerebellum develops from the rhombic lip and adjacent alar layer.

Adult neurogenesis

Until recently it was believed that no new neurones could be born in the adult mammalian brain; however, it is now clear that neural progenitor cells can be found in the adult CNS, including humans. These cells are predominantly found in parts of the hippocampus (see Chapter 45) and just next to the lateral ventricles in the subventricular zone (SVZ). They respond to a number of signals and appear to give rise to functional neurones in the hippocampus and olfactory bulb, with the latter cells migrating from the SVZ to the olfactory bulb via the rostral migratory stream (RMS).

Disorders of central nervous system embryogenesis

• *Anencephaly* occurs when there is failure of fusion of the anterior rostral neuropore. The cerebral vesicles fail to develop and thus there is no brain development. The vast majority of fetuses with this abnormality are spontaneously aborted.

• *Spina bifida* refers to any defect at the lower end of the vertebral column and/or spinal cord. The most common form of spina bifida refers to a failure of fusion of the dorsal parts of the lower vertebrae (*spina bifida occulta*). This can be associated with defects in the meninges and neural tissue which may herniate through the defect to form a *meningocoele* and *meningomyelocoele*, respectively. The most serious form of spina bifida is when nervous tissue is directly exposed as a result of a failure in the proper fusion of the posterior/caudal neuropore. Spina bifida is often associated with hydrocephalus (see Chapter 16).

Occasionally, bony defects are found at the base of the skull with the formation of a *meningocoele*. However, unlike the situation at the lower spinal cord, these can often be repaired without any neurological deficit being accrued.

• *Cortical dysplasia* refers to a spectrum of defects that are the result of the abnormal migration of developing cortical neurones. These defects are becoming increasingly recognized with improved imaging of the human CNS, and are now known to be an important cause of *epilepsy* (see Chapter 53).

• Many intrauterine infections (such as rubella), as well as some environmental agents (e.g. radiation), cause major problems in the development of the nervous system. In addition, a large number of rare genetic conditions are associated with defects of CNS development but these lie beyond the scope of this book.

3 The cells of the nervous system I: Neurones

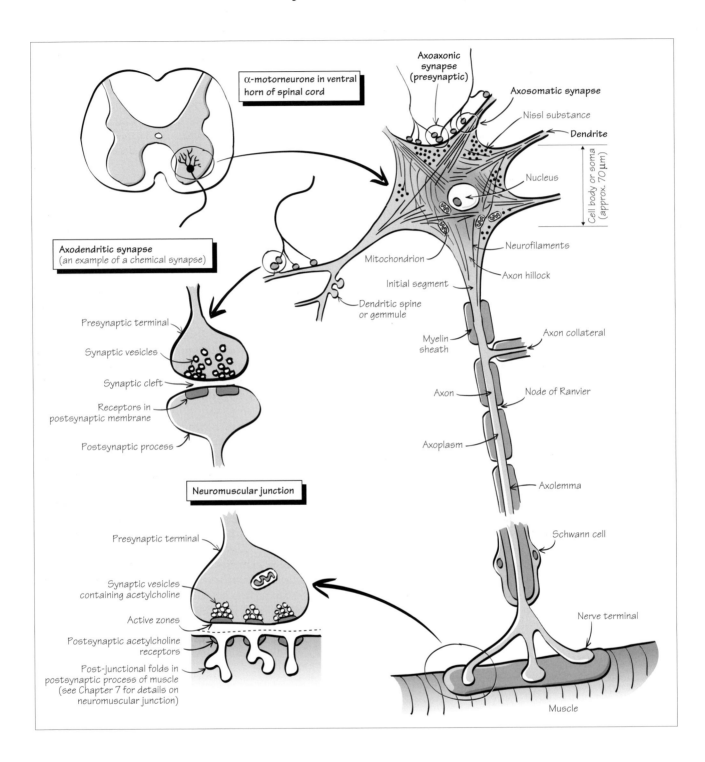

α-motorneurone in ventral horn of spinal cord

Axoaxonic synapse (presynaptic)

Axosomatic synapse

Nissl substance

Dendrite

Nucleus

Cell body or soma (approx. 70 μm)

Axodendritic synapse (an example of a chemical synapse)

Mitochondrion

Neurofilaments

Axon hillock

Initial segment

Dendritic spine or gemmule

Presynaptic terminal

Synaptic vesicles

Synaptic cleft

Receptors in postsynaptic membrane

Postsynaptic process

Myelin sheath

Axon collateral

Axon

Node of Ranvier

Axoplasm

Axolemma

Neuromuscular junction

Schwann cell

Presynaptic terminal

Synaptic vesicles containing acetylcholine

Active zones

Postsynaptic acetylcholine receptors

Post-junctional folds in postsynaptic process of muscle (see Chapter 7 for details on neuromuscular junction)

Nerve terminal

Muscle

There are two major classes of cells in the nervous system: the neuroglial cells and neurones, with the latter making up only 10–20% of the whole population. The neurones are specialized for excitation and nerve impulse conduction (see Chapters 5, 6 and 8), and communicate with each other by means of the synapse (see Chapter 7) and so act as the structural and functional unit of the nervous system.

Neurones

The **cell body (soma)** is that part of the neurone containing the nucleus and surrounding cytoplasm. It is the focus of cellular metabolism, and houses most of the neurone's intracellular organelles (**mitochondria**, Golgi apparatus and peroxisomes) and is associated typically with two types of neuronal process: the **dendrites** and **axon**. Most neurones also contain the granular basophilic staining, **Nissl substance**, which is composed of granular endoplasmic reticulum and ribosomes and is responsible for protein synthesis. This is located within the cell body and dendritic processes but is absent from the **axon hillock** and axon itself, for reasons that are not clear. In addition, throughout the cell body and processes are **neurofilaments** which are important in maintaining the architecture or cytoskeleton of the neurone. Furthermore, two other fibrillary structures within the neurone are important in this respect: microtubules and microfilaments, structures which are also important for axoplasmic flow (see below) and axonal growth.

The **dendrites** are neuronal cell processes that taper from the soma outwards, branch profusely and are responsible for conveying information towards the soma from **synapses** on the dendritic tree (**axodendritic synapses**; see also Chapter 8). Most neurones have many dendrites (**multipolar neurones**) and while some inputs synapse directly on the dendrite, some do so via small **dendritic spines or gemmules**. Thus, the primary role of dendrites is to increase the surface area for synapse formation allowing integration of a large number of inputs that are relayed to the cell body. In contrast, the **axon**, of which there is only one per neurone, conducts information away from the soma towards the **nerve terminal** and synapses (see Chapter 8). Although there is only one axon per neurone, it can branch to give several processes. This branching occurs close to the soma in the case of sensory neurones (**pseudo-unipolar** neurones; see Chapter 20), but more typically occurs close to the synaptic target of the axon. The axon originates from the soma at the **axon hillock** where the **initial segment** of the axon emerges. This is the most excitable part of a neurone because of its high density of sodium channels, and so is the site of initiation of the action potential (see Chapter 6).

All neurones are bounded by a lipid bilayer (**cell membrane**) within which proteins are located, some of which form ion channels (see Chapter 5), others form receptors to specific chemicals that are released by neurones (see Chapters 7 and 9) and others act as ion pumps moving ions across the membrane against their electrochemical gradient, e.g. Na^+–K^+ exchange pump (see Chapter 6). The axonal surface membrane is known as the **axolemma** and the cytoplasm contained within it, the **axoplasm**. The ion channels within the axolemma imbue the axon with its ability to conduct action potentials while the axoplasm contains neurofilaments, microtubules and mitochondria. These latter organelles are not only responsible for maintaining the ionic gradients necessary for action potential production but also allow for the transport and recycling of proteins away from (and to a lesser extent towards) the soma to the nerve terminal. This **axoplasmic flow or axonal transport** is either slow (~ 1 mm/day) or fast (~ 100–400 mm/day) and is not only important in permitting normal neuronal/synaptic activity but may also be important for neuronal survival and development and as such may be abnormal in some neurodegenerative disorders (see Chapter 52).

Many axons are surrounded by a layer of lipid, or **myelin sheath**, which acts as an electrical insulator. This myelin sheath alters the conducting properties of the axon, and allows for rapid action potential propagation without a loss of signal integrity (see Chapter 8). This is achieved by means of gaps, or **nodes (of Ranvier)**, in the myelin sheath where the axolemma contains many ion channels (typically Na^+ channels) which are directly exposed to the tissue fluid. The nodes of Ranvier are also those sites from which axonal branches originate, and these branches are termed **axon collaterals**. The myelin sheath encompasses the axon just beyond the initial segment and finishes just prior to its terminal arborization. The myelin sheath is formed by **Schwann cells** in the peripheral nervous system (PNS) and by **oligodendrocytes** in the central nervous system (CNS) (see Chapter 4), with many CNS axons being ensheathed by a single oligodendrocyte while in the PNS one Schwann cell provides myelin for one internode.

The **synapse** is the junction where a neurone meets another cell, which in the case of the CNS is another neurone. In the PNS the target can be muscle, glandular cells or other organs. The typical synapse in the nervous system is a **chemical** one, which is composed of a **presynaptic nerve terminal (bouton or end-bulb)** and a **synaptic cleft** which physically separates the nerve terminal from the **postsynaptic membrane** and across which the chemical or neurotransmitter from the presynaptic terminal must diffuse (see Chapter 7). This synapse is typically between an axon of one neurone and the dendrite of another (**axodendritic synapse**) although synapses are found where the point of contact between the axon and the postsynaptic cell is either at the level of the cell body (**axosomatic synapses**) or, less frequently, the presynaptic nerve terminal (**axoaxonic synapse**; see Chapter 8). A few synapses within the CNS do not possess these features but are low-resistance junctions (gap junctions) and are termed **electrical synapses**. These synapses allow for rapid conduction of action potentials without any integration and as such tend to enable populations of cells to fire together or in synchrony (see Chapters 7 and 53).

The specific loss of neurones is seen in a number of neurological disorders, and those diseases in which this is the primary event are discussed in Chapter 52.

4 The cells of the nervous system II: Neuroglial cells

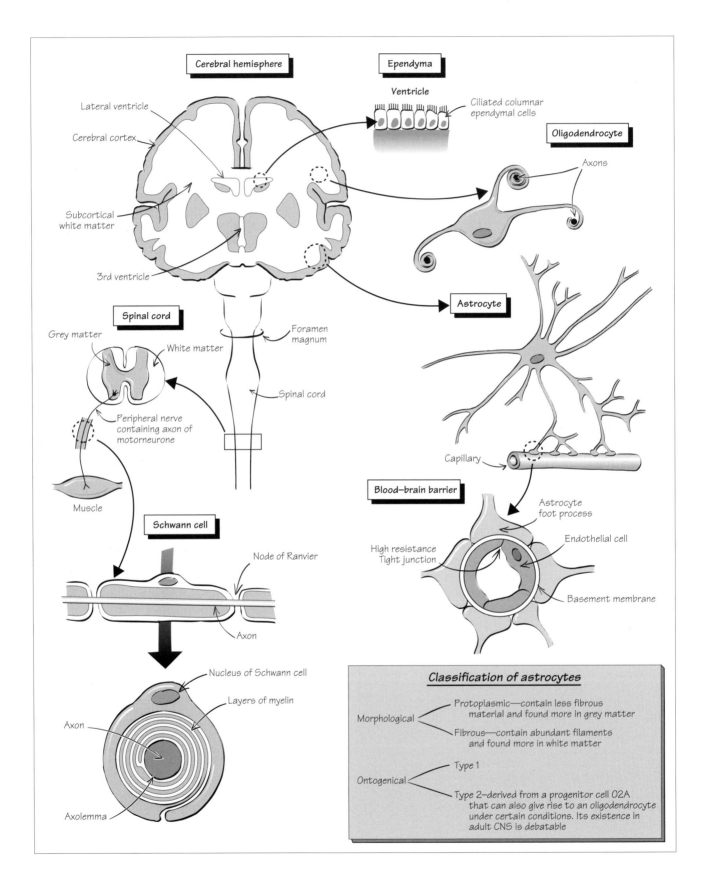

There are four main classes of neuroglial cells within the central nervous system (CNS): astrocytes, oligodendrocytes, ependymal cells and microglia, and they all subserve different functions. In contrast, in the peripheral nervous system (PNS), Schwann cells are the only example of neuroglia and are involved in myelination and facilitating axonal regeneration.

Astrocytes are small stellate cells that are found throughout the CNS and classified either morphologically or ontogenetically (see figure). They subserve many important functions within the CNS and are not simply passive support elements.

• They form a structural and supporting framework for neuronal cells and capillaries by virtue of their cytoplasmic processes, which end in close apposition not only to neurones but also capillaries. In this respect they form the glia limitans—where the astrocytic foot processes cover the basal laminae around blood vessels and at the pia mater.

• They maintain the integrity of the **blood–brain barrier (BBB)**, by promoting the formation of high-resistance junctions between brain capillary endothelial cells (see also Chapter 16).

• They are capable of taking up, storing and releasing some neurotransmitters (e.g. glutamate, γ-aminobutyric acid (GABA)) and thus may be an important adjunct in chemical neurotransmission within the CNS.

• They can take up and disperse excessive ion concentration in the extracellular fluid, especially K^+.

• They participate in neuronal guidance during development (see Chapter 15), and may also be important in the response to injury (see Chapter 47) and in the fate of neural precursor cells in the adult hippocampus.

• They may have a role in presenting antigen to the immune system in situations where the CNS and BBB are damaged (see Chapter 54).

The most common clinical disorder of astrocytes is their abnormal proliferation in tumours called ***astrocytomas***. These tumours produce effects by compressing adjacent CNS tissue and this presents as an evolving neurological deficit (with or without epileptic seizures) depending on its site of origin within the CNS. In adults, the tumours most commonly arise in the white matter of the cerebral hemispheres.

Oligodendrocytes are responsible for the myelination of CNS neurones, and are therefore found in large numbers in the white matter. Each oligodendrocyte forms internodal myelin for 3–50 fibres and also surrounds many other fibres without forming myelin sheaths. In addition, they have a number of molecules associated with them that are inhibitory to axonal growth, and thus contribute to the failure of damaged adult CNS neurones to regenerate (see Chapter 47).

Clinical disorders of oligodendrocyte function cause central demyelination which is seen in a number of conditions including ***multiple sclerosis*** (see Chapter 54), while abnormal proliferation of oligodendrocytes produces a slow-growing tumour (an ***oligodendroglioma***) which tends to present with epileptic seizures (see Chapter 53).

Ependymal cells are important in facilitating the movement of cerebrospinal fluid (CSF) as well as interacting with astrocytes to form a barrier separating the ventricles and the CSF from the neuronal environment. They also line the central canal in the spinal cord (see Chapter 12). These ependymal cells are termed ependymocytes to distinguish them from those ependymal cells that are involved in the formation of CSF (the choroid plexus) and those that transport substances from the CSF to blood (tanycytes). Tumours of the ependyma (***ependymomas or choroid plexus papillomas***) occur either in the ventricles where they tend to produce ***hydrocephalus*** (see Chapter 16) or spinal cord where they cause local destruction of the neural structures.

Microglial cells (not shown on figure) are the tissue macrophages of the brain, and are found throughout the white and grey matter of the CNS. They are phagocytic in nature and are important in mediating immune responses within the CNS (see Chapter 54).

Schwann cells are found only in the PNS and are responsible for the myelination of peripheral nerves by a process that involves the wrapping of the cell around the axon. Thus, the final myelin sheath is composed of multiple layers of Schwann cell membrane in which the cytoplasm has been extruded. Unlike oligodendrocytes, one Schwann cell envelops one axon and provides myelin for one internode. In addition, Schwann cells are important in the regeneration of damaged peripheral axons, in contrast to the largely inhibitory functions of the central neuroglial cells (see Chapters 46 and 47). A number of genetic and inflammatory neuropathies are associated with the loss of peripheral myelin (as opposed to the loss of axons), which results in peripheral nerve dysfunction (***demyelinating neuropathies***; see Chapters 6 and 55). In addition, benign tumours of Schwann cells can occur (***schwannomas***), especially in certain genetic conditions such as ***neurofibromatosis type I***, where there is the loss of the tumour suppressor gene, neurofibromin. These tumours are typically asymptomatic but if they arise in areas of limited space they can produce symptoms by compression of the neighbouring neural structures; for example, at the cerebellopontine angle in the brainstem or spinal root (see Chapters 12–14 and 27).

5 Ion channels

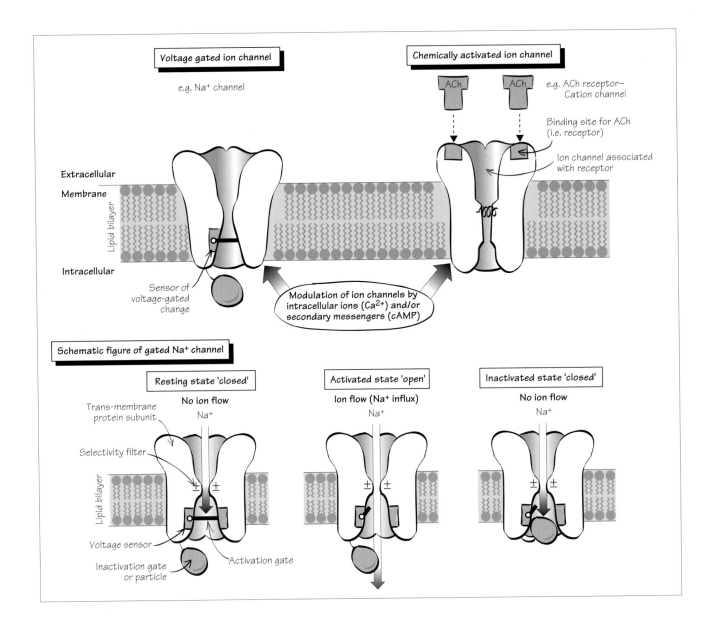

Voltage gated ion channel

e.g. Na⁺ channel

Chemically activated ion channel

e.g. ACh receptor–Cation channel

Binding site for ACh (i.e. receptor)

Ion channel associated with receptor

Extracellular

Membrane

Lipid bilayer

Intracellular

Sensor of voltage-gated change

Modulation of ion channels by intracellular ions (Ca²⁺) and/or secondary messengers (cAMP)

Schematic figure of gated Na⁺ channel

Trans-membrane protein subunit

Selectivity filter

Lipid bilayer

Voltage sensor

Inactivation gate or particle

Activation gate

Resting state 'closed'

No ion flow
Na⁺

Activated state 'open'

Ion flow (Na⁺ influx)
Na⁺

Inactivated state 'closed'

No ion flow
Na⁺

An **ion channel** is a protein macromolecule that spans a biological membrane and allows ions to pass from one side of the membrane to the other. The ions move in a direction determined by the electrochemical gradient across the membrane. In general, ions will tend to flow from an area of high concentration to one of low concentration, but in the presence of a voltage gradient it is possible for there to be no ion flow even with unequal concentrations. The ion channel itself can be open or closed. Opening can be achieved either by changing the voltage across the membrane (e.g. a depolarization or the arrival of an action potential) or by the binding of a chemical substance to a receptor in or near the channel. The two types of channel are called **voltage gated** (or **voltage sensitive**) and **chemically activated** (or **ligand gated**) channels, respectively. However, this distinction is somewhat artificial as a number of voltage sensitive channels can be modulated by neurotransmitters as well as by Ca²⁺. Furthermore, some ion channels are not

opened by voltage changes or chemical messengers but are directly opened by mechanical stretch or pressure (e.g. the somatosensory and auditory receptors; see Chapters 19, 20 and 26).

The most important property of ion channels is that they imbue the neurone with electrical excitability (see Chapter 6) and while they are found in all parts of the neurone, and to a lesser extent in neuroglial cells, they are also seen in a host of non-neural cells.

All biological membranes, including the neuronal membrane, are composed of a lipid bilayer that has a high electrical resistance, i.e. ions will not readily flow through it. Therefore in order for ions to move across a membrane it is necessary to have either 'pores' (ion channels) in the lipid bilayer or 'carriers' that will collect the ions from one side of the membrane and carry them across to the other side where they are released. In neurones the rate of ion transfer necessary for signal transmission is too fast for any carrier system and so ion channels (or 'pores') are employed by neurones for the transfer of ions across the membrane.

The fundamental properties of an ion channel are as follows:
• It is composed of a number of protein subunits that traverse the membrane and allow ions to cross from one side to the other—a **transmembrane pore**.
• The channel so formed must be able to move from a **closed** to an **open** state and back, although intermediate steps may be required.
• It must be able to open in response to specific stimuli. Most channels possess a sensor of voltage change and so open in response to a depolarizing voltage, i.e. one that moves the resting membrane potential from its resting value of $-70\,mV$ to a less negative value.

In contrast, some channels, especially those found at synapses, are not opened by a voltage change but by a chemical, e.g. acetylcholine (ACh). These channels have a **receptor** for that chemical and the binding of the chemical to this receptor leads to channel opening. However, many channels possess both voltage and chemical sensors and the presence of an intracellular ion or secondary messenger molecule (e.g. cyclic adenosine monophosphate (cAMP)) leads to a **modulation** of the ion flow across the membrane which the voltage-dependent process has produced.

Activation of the voltage sensor or chemical receptor leads to the opening of a **'gate'** within the channel which allows ions to flow through the channel. The channel is then closed by either a process of **deactivation** (which is simply the reversal of the opening of the gate) or **inactivation** which involves a **second gate** moving into the channel more slowly than the activation gate moves out, so that there is a time when there is no gate in the channel and ions can flow through it.

The flow of ions through the channel can be either **selective or non-selective**. If the channel is selective then it only allows certain ions through and it achieves this by means of a **'filter'**. The selectivity filter is based on energetic considerations (thermodynamically) and gives the channel its name, e.g. the sodium channel. However, certain channels are non-selective in that they allow many different types of similarly charged ions through, e.g. the ACh cation channel.

The overall description of an ion channel is in terms of a number of different physical measures. The net flow of ions through a channel is termed the **current**; while the **conductance** is defined as the reciprocal of resistance (current/voltage) and represents the ease with which the ions can pass through the membrane. **Permeability**, on the other hand, is defined as the rate of transport of a substance or ion through the membrane for a given concentration difference.

There are many different types of ion channels and even within a single family of ion-specific channels there are multiple subtypes, e.g. there are at least five different types of potassium channels.

The number and type of ion channels governs the response characteristics of the cell. In the case of neurones, this is expressed in terms of the rate of action potential generation and its response to synaptic inputs (see Chapters 6–8, 45 and 53).

Clinical disorders of ion channels

A number of pharmacological agents work at the level of ion channels, including local anaesthetics and some antiepileptic drugs. However, in recent years a number of neurological disorders, primarily involving muscle, have been found to be caused by mutations in the sodium and chloride ion channels. These conditions include various forms of *myotonia* (delayed relaxation of skeletal muscle following voluntary contraction, i.e. an inability to let go of objects easily) and various forms of *periodic paralyses* in which patients develop a transient flaccid weakness which can be either partial or generalized. Furthermore, certain forms of familial hemiplegic *migraine* and cerebellar dysfunction (see Chapter 37) are associated with abnormalities in the Ca^{2+} channel, and some forms of *epilepsy* (see Chapter 53) may be caused by a disorder of specific ion channels. In other disorders there is a redistribution or exposing of normally non-functioning ion channels. This commonly occurs next to the node of Ranvier as a result of central demyelination in *multiple sclerosis* and peripheral demyelination in the *Guillain–Barré syndrome*, and results in an impairment in action potential propagation (see Chapters 6 and 54).

6 The resting membrane and action potential

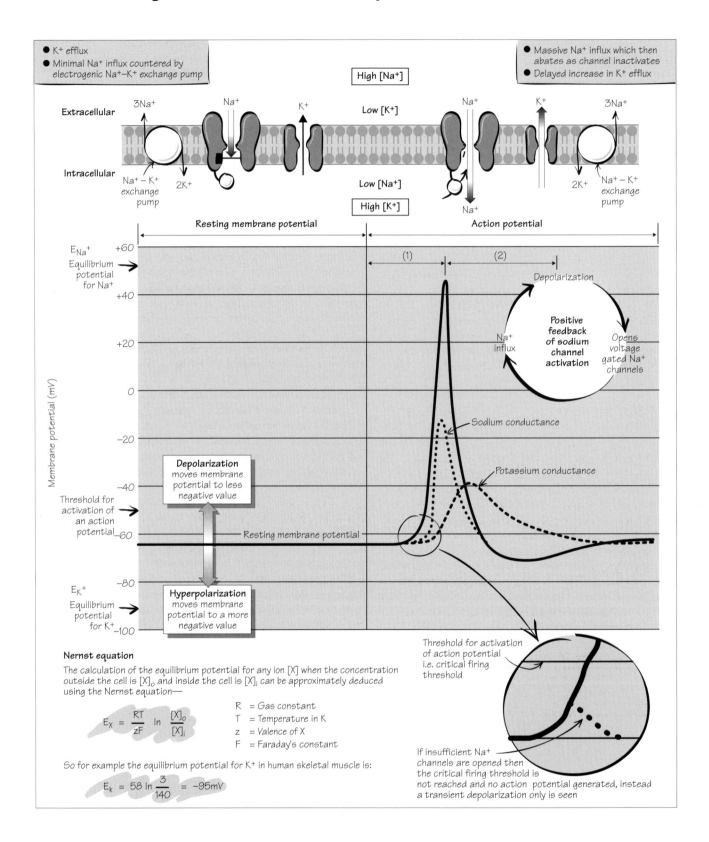

Nernst equation

The calculation of the equilibrium potential for any ion [X] when the concentration outside the cell is $[X]_o$ and inside the cell is $[X]_i$ can be approximately deduced using the Nernst equation—

$$E_X = \frac{RT}{zF} \ln \frac{[X]_o}{[X]_i}$$

R = Gas constant
T = Temperature in K
z = Valence of X
F = Faraday's constant

So for example the equilibrium potential for K+ in human skeletal muscle is:

$$E_k = 58 \ln \frac{3}{140} = -95mV$$

Resting membrane potential

In the resting state the neuronal cell membrane is relatively impermeable to ions. This is important in the generation of the **resting membrane potential**. The major intracellular ion is potassium compared to sodium in the extracellular fluid and so the natural flow of ions according to their concentration gradients is for K^+ to leave the cell (or efflux) and for Na^+ to enter (or influx). The movement of positive ions out of the cell leads to the generation of a negative membrane potential or **hyperpolarization**, while the converse is true for positive ion influx (a process of **depolarization**). However, the resting membrane is relatively impermeable to Na^+ ions while being relatively permeable to K^+ ions. At rest therefore, K^+ will tend to efflux from the cell down its concentration gradient leaving excess negative charge behind and this will continue until the chemical concentration gradient driving K^+ out of the cell is exactly offset by the electrical potential difference generated by this efflux (the membrane potential) drawing K^+ back into the cell. The membrane potential at which this steady state is achieved is the **equilibrium potential** for K^+ (E_{K^+}) and can be derived using the **Nernst equation** (see figure for details). In fact the measured resting membrane potential in axons is slightly more positive than expected because there is some small permeability to Na^+ of the membrane in the resting state. The small Na^+ influx is countered by an adenosine triphosphate (ATP) dependent **Na^+–K^+ exchange pump** which is itself slightly electrogenic. This pump is essential in maintaining the ionic gradients, and is electrogenic by virtue of the fact that it pumps out three Na^+ ions for every two K^+ ions brought in. It makes only a small contribution to the level of the resting membrane potential.

Action potential generation

One of the fundamental features of the nervous system is its ability to generate and conduct electrical impulses (see Chapters 8 and 19). These can take the form of generator potentials, synaptic potentials and action potentials—the latter being defined as a single electrical impulse passing down an axon. **This action potential (nerve impulse or spike) is an all or nothing phenomenon**, that is to say once the threshold stimulus intensity is reached an action potential will be generated. Therefore information in the nervous system is coded by frequency of firing rather than size of the action potential (see Chapter 18). The threshold stimulus intensity is defined as that value at which the net inward current (which is largely determined by Na^+ ions) is just greater than the net outward current (which is largely carried by K^+ ions), and is typically around $-55\,mV$ (**critical firing threshold**). This occurs most readily in the region of the axon hillock where there is the highest density of Na^+ channels, and is thus the site of action potential initiation in the neurone. However, if the threshold is not reached the graded depolarization will not generate an action potential and the signal will not be propagated along the axon.

The sequence of events in the generation of an action potential are as follows:

(1) The depolarizing voltage activates the voltage sensitive Na^+ channels in the neuronal membrane which allows some Na^+ ions to flow down their electrochemical gradient (increased Na^+ conductance). This depolarizes the membrane still further opening more Na^+ channels in a **positive feedback loop**. When sufficient Na^+ channels are opened to produce an inward current greater than that generated by the K^+ efflux, there is rapid opening of all the Na^+ channels producing a large influx of Na^+ which depolarizes the membrane towards the **equilibrium potential for Na^+** ($\sim +55\,mV$). The spike of the action potential is therefore generated, but fails to reach the equilibrium potential for Na^+ because of the persistent and increasing K^+ efflux.

(2) The falling phase of the action potential then follows as the voltage sensitive Na^+ channels become inactivated (see Chapter 5). This inactivation is voltage dependent, in that it is in response to the depolarizing stimulus, but has slower kinetics than the activation process and so occurs later (see also Chapter 5). During this falling phase a voltage dependent K^+ current becomes important as its activation by the depolarization of the membrane has even slower kinetics than sodium channel inactivation. This voltage activated K^+ channel leads to a brief period of membrane hyperpolarization before it deactivates and the membrane potential is returned to the resting state.

Immediately after the spike of the action potential there is a **refractory period** when the neurone is either inexcitable (**absolute refractory period**) or only activated to submaximal responses by suprathreshold stimuli (**relative refractory period**). The absolute refractory period occurs at the time of maximal Na^+ channel inactivation while the relative refractory period occurs at a later time when most of the Na^+ channels have returned to their resting state but the voltage activated K^+ current is well developed. The refractory period has two important implications for action potential generation and conduction. First, action potentials can be conducted only in one direction, away from the site of its generation and, secondly, they can be generated only up to certain limiting frequencies (see Chapter 18).

The original description of the mechanism of generation of the action potential was by Hodgkin and Huxley in the squid giant axon in the 1950s but subsequently has been confirmed in many other cells and neurones. This, together with the discovery of a large number of ion channels, has meant that many modifications relating to the generation and characteristics of action potentials in neurones and other cells have been described.

7 The neuromuscular junction and synapses

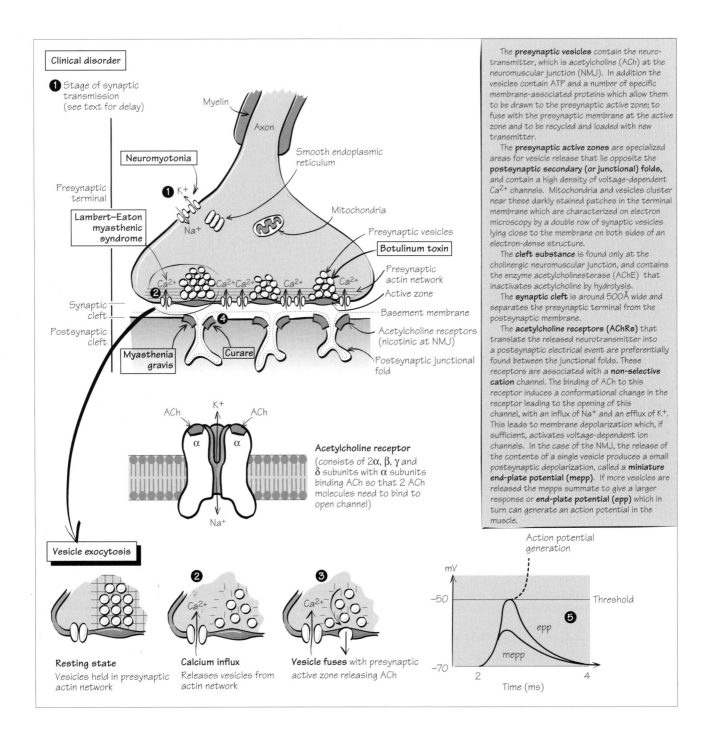

Sherrington in 1897 coined the term **'synapse'** to mean the junction of two neurones. Much of the work on the synapse has been done with the cholinergic **neuromuscular junction (NMJ)**, although it appears that this chemical synapse is similar in its mode of action to those found in the central nervous system (CNS). The chemical synapse is the predominant synapse type found in the nervous system, but electrical synapses are found in certain sites, e.g. glial cells (see also Chapter 4).

Neuromuscular transmission (a model for synaptic transmission)

The sequence of events at a chemical synapse is as follows:
• The arrival of the action potential leads to the depolarization of the presynaptic terminal (labelled (**1**) on figure) with the opening of **voltage-dependent Ca^{2+} channels** in the **active zones** of the presynaptic terminal and subsequent Ca^{2+} influx (**2**) (this is the stage that represents the major delay in synaptic transmission).

• The influx of Ca^{2+} leads to the phosphorylation and alteration of a number of presynaptic calcium-binding proteins (some of which are found in the vesicle membrane) which liberates the **vesicle** from its **presynaptic actin network** allowing it to bind to the **presynaptic membrane (3)**. These proteins include various different soluble NSF attachment proteins (SNAPs) and SNAP receptors (SNAREs).

• The fusion of the two hemichannels (presynaptic vesicle and presynaptic membrane) leads to the formation of a small pore that rapidly expands with the release of vesicular contents into the **synaptic cleft**. The vesicle membrane can then be recycled by **endocytosis** into the presynaptic terminal, either by a non-selective or more selective clathrin-mediated process.

• Most of the released neurotransmitter then diffuses across the synaptic cleft and binds to the **postsynaptic receptor (4)**. Some transmitter molecules diffuse out of the synaptic cleft and are lost, while others are inactivated before they have time to bind to the postsynaptic membrane receptor. This **inactivation** is essential for the synapse to function normally and, although enzymatic degradation of acetylcholine (ACh) is employed at the NMJ, other synapses employ uptake mechanisms with the recycling of the transmitter into the presynaptic neurone (see Chapter 9).

• The activation of the postsynaptic receptor leads to a change in the postsynaptic membrane potential. Each vesicle contains a certain amount or quantum of neurotransmitter, whose release generates a small postsynaptic potential change of a fixed size—the **miniature end-plate potential (mepp)**. The release of transmitter from several vesicles leads to mepp summation and the generation of a larger depolarization or **end-plate potential (epp)** which, if sufficiently large, will reach threshold for action potential generation in the postsynaptic muscle fibre **(5)**.

This **vesicle hypothesis** has been criticized, because not all CNS synapses contain their neurotransmitters in vesicles and because electrical synapses are found in some neural networks. Alternative theories have therefore been put forward that invoke either molecules to carry the neurotransmitter across the presynaptic membrane or pores that open in the presynaptic membrane in response to a calcium influx. There is little evidence in favour of either of these theories.

Disorders of neuromuscular transmission

There are a number of naturally occurring toxins that can affect the NMJ.

• **Curare** binds to the acetylcholine receptor (AChR) and prevents ACh from acting on it and so induces paralysis. This is exploited clinically in the use of curare derivatives for muscle paralysis in certain forms of surgery.

• **Botulinum toxin** prevents the release of ACh presynaptically. In this case an exotoxin from the bacterium *Clostridium botulinum* binds to the presynaptic membrane of the ACh synapse and prevents the quantal release of ACh. The accidental ingestion of this toxin in cases of food poisoning produces paralysis and autonomic failure (see Chapter 42). However, the toxin can be used therapeutically in small quantities by injecting it into muscles that are abnormally overactive in certain forms of focal *dystonia*—a condition in which a part of the body is held in a fixed abnormal posture by overactive muscular activity (see Chapter 39).

A number of neurological conditions affect the NMJ selectively. These include ***myasthenia gravis, the Lambert–Eaton myasthenic syndrome (LEMS)*** and ***neuromyotonia or Isaac's syndrome***. In ***neuromyotonia*** the patient complains of muscle cramps and stiffness as a result of continuous motor activity in the muscle. This is often caused by an antibody directed against the presynaptic voltage-gated K^+ channel, so the nerve terminal is always in a state of depolarization with transmitter release. In contrast, in ***LEMS*** there is an antibody directed against the presynaptic Ca^{2+} channel, so that on repeated activation of the synapse there is a steady increase in Ca^{2+} influx as the blocking antibody is competitively overcome by exogenous Ca^{2+}. The patient complains of weakness, especially of the proximal muscles, which transiently improves on exercise. ***Myasthenia gravis***, on the other hand, is caused by an antibody against the AChR, and patients complain of weakness that increases with exercise (fatiguability) involving the eyes, throat and limbs. This weakness is because the number of AChR are reduced and the presynaptic release of ACh competes for the few available receptors.

Electrical synapses

Electrical transmission occurs at a small number of sites in the brain. The presence of fast conducting gap junctions promotes the rapid and widespread propagation of electrical activity and thus may be important in synchronizing some aspects of cortical function (see Chapter 15). The abnormal absence of gap junctions in Schwann cells leads to one form of peripheral hereditary motor sensory neuropathy (HMSN).

8 Nerve conduction and synaptic integration

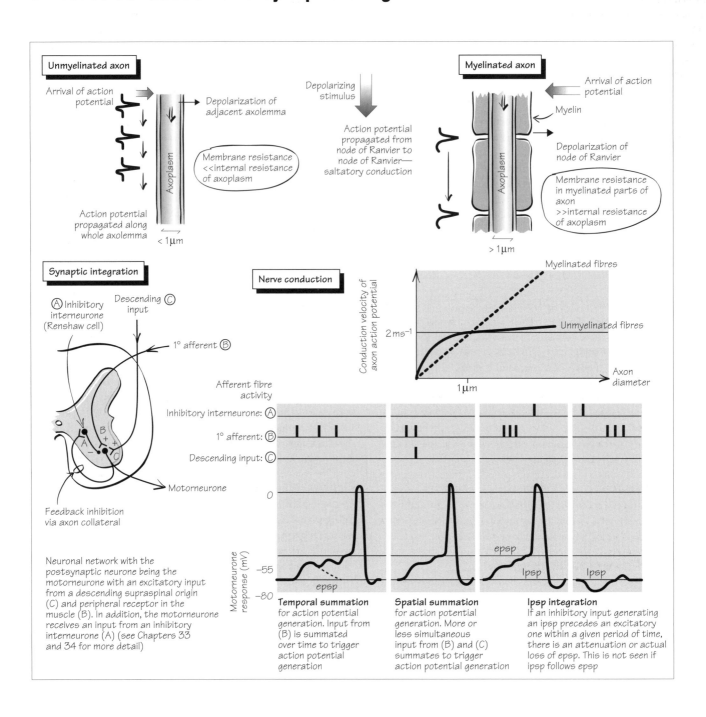

Nerve conduction

Action potential propagation is achieved by local current spread and is made possible by the large safety factor in the generation of an action potential as a consequence of the positive feedback of Na^+ channel activation in the rising phase of the nerve impulse (see Chapter 6). The use of local current spread does, however, set constraints not only on the velocity of nerve conduction but also influences the fidelity of the signal being conducted. The nervous system overcomes these difficulties by insulating nerve fibres above a given diameter with myelin which is periodically interrupted by the nodes of Ranvier.

In **unmyelinated axons** an action potential at one site leads to depolarization of the membrane immediately in front and theoretically behind it, although the membrane at this site is in its refractory state and so the action potential is only conducted in one direction (see Chapter 6). The current preferentially passes across the membrane (because of the high internal resistance of the axoplasm) and is greatest at the site closest to the action potential.

However, while nerve impulse conduction is feasible and accurate in unmyelinated axons, especially in the very small diameter fibres where the internal axoplasmic resistance is very high, it is nevertheless slow.

Conduction velocity can therefore be increased by either increasing the axon diameter (of which the best example is the squid giant axon with a diameter of ~1 mm) or insulating the axon using a high-resistance substance such as the lipid-rich myelin.

Conduction in **myelinated fibres** follows exactly the same sequence of events as in unmyelinated fibres, but with a crucial difference; the advancing action potential encounters a high-resistance low-capacitance structure in the form of a nerve fibre wrapped in myelin. The depolarizing current therefore passes along the axoplasm until it reaches a low-resistance **node of Ranvier** with its high density of Na^+ channels and an action potential is generated at this site. The action potential therefore appears to be conducted down the fibre, from node to node—a process termed **saltatory conduction**. The advantage of myelination is that it allows for rapid conduction while minimizing the metabolic demands on the cell. It also increases the packing capacity of the nervous system, so that many fast conducting fibres can be packed into a small nerve. As a result most axons over a certain diameter (~1 μm) are myelinated.

Disturbances in nerve conduction are clinically seen when there is a disruption of the myelin sheath, e.g. in the peripheral nervous system (PNS) in inflammatory demyelinating neuropathies such as the *Guillain–Barré syndrome* and in the central nervous system (CNS) with *multiple sclerosis* (see Chapter 54). In both conditions there is a loss of the myelin sheath, especially in the area adjacent to the node of Ranvier, which exposes other ion channels, as well as reducing the length of insulation along the axon. The result is that the propagated action potential has to depolarize a greater area of axolemma, part of which is not as excitable as the normal node of Ranvier because it contains fewer Na^+ channels. This leads to slowing of the action potential propagation and, if the demyelination is severe enough, actually leads to an attenuation of the propagated action potential to the point that it can no longer be conducted—so-called conduction block.

Synaptic integration

Each central neurone receives many hundreds of synapses and each input is integrated into a response by that neurone, a process that involves the summation of inputs from many different sites at any one time (**spatial summation**) as well as the summation of one or several inputs over time (**temporal summation**).

The presynaptic nerve terminal usually contains one neurotransmit-ter, although the release of two or more transmitters at a single presynaptic terminal has been described—a process termed **cotransmission** (see Chapter 9). The amount of neurotransmitter released is dependent not only on the degree to which the presynaptic terminal is depolarized but also the rate of neurotransmitter synthesis, the presence of inhibitory presynaptic autoreceptors and presynaptic inputs from other neurones in the form of axoaxonic synapses (see Chapter 3). These synapses are usually inhibitory (presynaptic inhibition) and are more common in sensory pathways (see, for example, Chapter 18).

The released neurotransmitter acts on a specific protein or **receptor** in the postsynaptic membrane and in certain synapses on **presynaptic autoreceptors** (see Chapter 9). When this binding leads to an opening of ion channels with a cation influx in the postsynaptic process with depolarization, then the synapse is said to be **excitatory**, while those ion channels that allow postsynaptic anion influx or cation efflux with hyperpolarization are termed **inhibitory**.

Excitatory postsynaptic potentials (EPSPs) are the depolarizations recorded in the postsynaptic cell to a given excitatory synaptic input. The depolarizations associated with the EPSPs can go on to induce action potentials if they are summated either in time or space. **Spatial summation** involves the integration by the postsynaptic cell of several EPSPs at different synapses with the summed depolarization being sufficient to induce an action potential. **Temporal summation**, on the other hand, involves the summation of inputs in time such that each successive EPSP depolarizes the membrane still further until the threshold for action potential generation is reached. In contrast, **inhibitory postsynaptic potentials (IPSPs)** are hyperpolarizations of the postsynaptic membrane, usually as a result of an influx of Cl^- and an efflux of K^+ through their respective ion channels. IPSPs are very important in modulating the neurone's response to excitatory synaptic inputs (see figure). Therefore inhibitory synapses tend to be found in strategically important sites on the neurone—the proximal dendrite and soma—so that they can have profound effects on the input from large parts of the dendritic tree. In addition, some neurones can inhibit their own output by the use of axon collaterals and a local inhibitory interneurone (**feedback inhibition**), e.g. motorneurones and Renshaw cells of the spinal cord (see Chapter 34).

More **long-term modulations of synaptic transmission** are discussed in Chapters 37, 45 and 53.

9 Neurotransmitters, receptors and their pathways

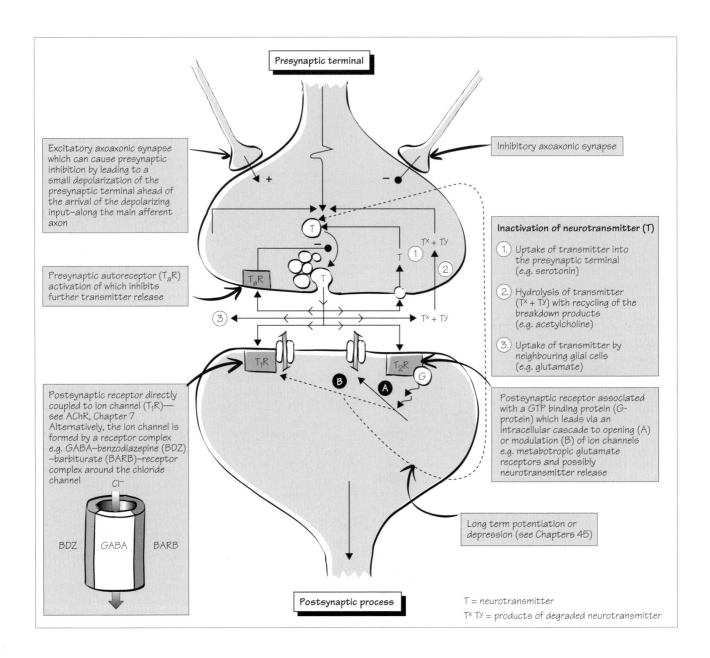

Neurotransmitters and synaptic function

The neurotransmitter released at a synapse interacts with a specific protein in the postsynaptic membrane, known as a **receptor**. At some synapses the neurotransmitter also binds to a **presynaptic autoreceptor** that regulates the amount of transmitter that is released. Receptors are usually specific for a given neurotransmitter, although several different types of that receptor may exist. In some cases coreleased neurotransmitters can either modulate the binding of another neurotransmitter to its receptor or act synergistically on a common single ion channel (e.g. the **γ-aminobutyric acid (GABA)–benzodiazepine–barbiturate receptor**).

Receptors for specific neurotransmitters are either **coupled directly to ion channels** (T_1R on figure, e.g. acetylcholine receptors (AChR);

see Chapter 7) or **to a membrane enzyme (T_2R)**. In these latter instances the binding of the neurotransmitter to the receptor either opens an ion channel via an intracellular enzyme cascade (e.g. cyclic adenosine monophosphate (cAMP) and G-proteins) or indirectly modulates the probability of other ion channels opening in response to voltage changes (**neuromodulation**). These receptors therefore mediate slower synaptic events, unlike those receptors directly coupled to ion channels that relay fast synaptic information.

The activated receptor can only return to its resting state once the neurotransmitter has been removed either by a process of enzymatic **hydrolysis** or **uptake** into the presynaptic nerve terminal or neighbouring glial cells. Even then there are often intermediate steps in the process of returning the receptor and its associated ion channel to the resting state. At some synapses the affinity and, ultimately, the number of receptors is dependent on the previous activity of the synapse. For example, at catecholaminergic synapses the receptors become less sensitive to the released transmitter when the synapse is very active — a process of **desensitization and down-regulation**. This process involves a decrease in the affinity of the receptor for the transmitter in the short term, which goes on in the long term to an actual decrease in the number of receptors.

The converse is true with synapses that are rarely activated (**supersensitivity and up-regulation**), and in this way synaptic activity is modulated by its ongoing activity. In addition, at some synapses the activation of the postsynaptic receptor–ion channel complex can modulate the long-term activity of the synapse, either by affecting the presynaptic release of neurotransmitter or the postsynaptic receptor response — a process known as either **long-term potentiation (LTP) or long-term depression (LTD)** depending on the actual change in synaptic efficacy over time (see Chapters 37 and 45).

Therefore the state, number and types of receptors for a specific neurotransmitter as well as the presence of receptors to other neurotransmitters are all important in determining the extent of synaptic activity at any given synapse.

Diversity and anatomy of neurotransmitter pathways

The nervous system employs a large number of neurotransmitters, but these can be seen to form families (see Appendix 1).

Excitatory amino acids

These represent the main excitatory neurotransmitters in the central nervous system (CNS) and are important at most synapses in maintaining ongoing synaptic activity. The main excitatory amino acid is **glutamate** which acts at a number of receptors, which are defined by the agonists that activate them. The **ionotropic** receptors consist of the *N*-**methyl-D-aspartate (NMDA)** and **non-NMDA receptors**, and the former receptor with its associated calcium channel may be important in the generation of LTP (see Chapter 45), excitotoxic cell death (see Chapter 52) and possibly *epilepsy* (see Chapter 53).

A separate group of G-protein associated glutamate receptors, the **metabotropic receptors**, respond on activation by initiating a number of intracellular biochemical events that modulate synaptic transmission and neuronal activity. These receptors may underlie long-term depression in the hippocampus.

Inhibitory amino acids

The major CNS inhibitory neurotransmitters are **GABA**, which is present throughout the CNS, and **glycine** which is predominantly found in the spinal cord. Abnormalities of GABA neurones may underlie some forms of movement disorders as well as anxiety states and epilepsy (see Chapters 42, 51 and 53) while mutations in the glycine receptor have now been linked to some forms of *hyperekplexia* — a condition in which there is an excessive startle response, such that any stimulus induces a stiffening of the body with collapse to the ground without any impairment of consciousness.

Monoamines

The monoaminergic systems of the CNS originate from small groups of neurones in the brainstem, which then project widely to all areas of the CNS. They are found at many other sites within the body, including the autonomic nervous system (see Chapter 42). In all locations they bind to a host of different receptors and thus can have complex actions (see Chapters 21, 38 and 45).

Acetylcholine

This neurotransmitter is widely distributed throughout the nervous system, including the neuromuscular junction (see Chapter 7) and autonomic nervous system (see Chapter 42). Therefore, many agents have been developed that target the different cholinergic synapses in the periphery and which are used routinely in surgical anaesthesia. Several disease processes can affect the peripherally located cholinergic synapses (see Chapter 7), while secondary abnormalities in the central cholinergic pathways may be important in *Parkinson's disease and dementia of the Alzheimer type* (see Chapters 39 and 52).

Neuropeptides

These neurotransmitters, of which there are many different types, are found in all areas of the nervous system and are often coreleased with other neurotransmitters. They can act as conventional neurotransmitters as well as having a role in neuromodulation (e.g. pain pathways, see Chapters 21 and 22).

10 Skeletal muscle structure

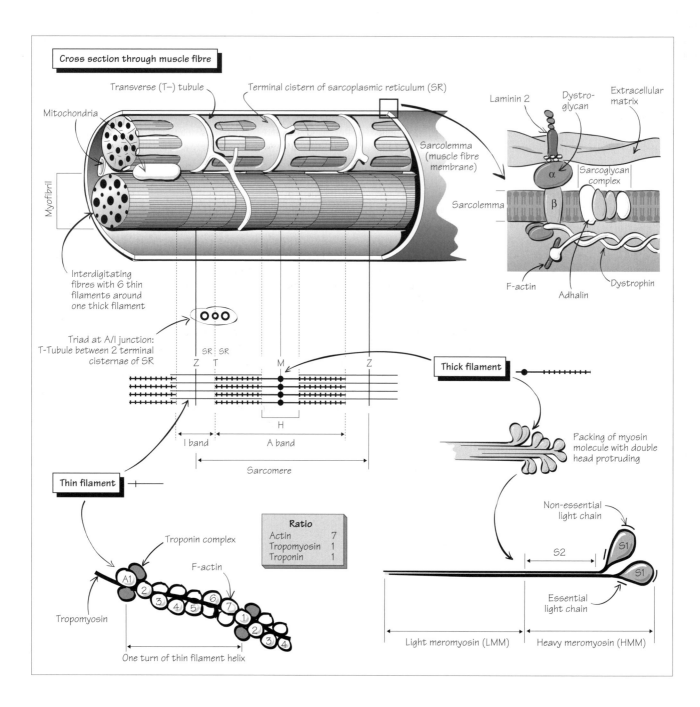

Skeletal muscle is responsible for converting the electrical impulse from a lower motorneurone that arrives at the neuromuscular junction (NMJ) into a mechanical force by means of contraction. The arrival of the action potential leads to the release of acetylcholine (ACh) which activates the nicotinic ACh receptor (AChR) in the postsynaptic muscle, which in turn leads to the depolarization of the muscle fibre (see Chapter 7). This produces a calcium influx into the muscle fibre which leads to muscle contraction (see Chapter 11).

Structure of skeletal muscle

Skeletal muscle is composed of groups of muscle fibres which are long,

multinucleated cells. These fibres contain **myofibrils**, which in turn are made up of thick and thin filaments that overlap to some extent giving this type of muscle its striated appearance. The myofibrils are bounded by the **sarcolemma** which invaginates amongst the myofibrils in the form of **transverse or T-tubules**. This structure is separate from the **sarcoplasmic reticulum (SR)** which envelops the myofibrils and is important as an intracellular store of Ca^{2+}. The sarcolemma is a complex structure and abnormalities in some of its membrane components have recently been found to underlie some forms of inherited muscular dystrophies.

The **thick filament** is composed of myosin and lies at the centre of the **sarcomere**. Myosin is composed of two heavy chains that form the **light and heavy meromyosin proteins** (LMM and HMM, respectively). The HMM portion contains **S1 and S2 subfragments**. The S1 fragment consists of two heads and associated with each head are two light chains. The light chain found at the tip of the S1 head is termed **non-essential** and is responsible for breaking down adenosine triphosphate (ATP) at the end of the power stroke of crossbridge formation. The remaining **essential** light chain is attached at the point where the S1 head swings out towards the actin and is important in the process of myosin head movement. By virtue of the properties of LMM, myosin filaments spontaneously pack together so that the S1 heads are on the outside towards the actin filaments. The S1 heads therefore form the major part of the crossbridge with the actin.

Thin filaments are composed of **F-actin, tropomyosin and troponin**, which is itself composed of three subunits (troponin-I, -C and -T). These three components of the troponin complex all subserve different functions but as a whole they regulate muscle contraction by holding the tropomyosin in position so that it physically blocks the S1 head of the myosin from binding to the actin. The depolarization of the muscle leads to a calcium influx which then binds to troponin, producing a conformational change in the thin filament such that the tropomyosin shifts off the binding site for myosin on actin. Thus, tropomyosin and troponin regulate muscle contraction by a process of **stearic block**. In some muscles in other animals the regulation of the interaction between actin and myosin lies with the myosin-associated light chains.

At the point of overlap of these two sets of filaments the **triad** structure of a T-tubule linked to two terminal cisternae of SR by foot processes is to be found.

Disorders of structural proteins in skeletal muscle — the muscular dystrophies

There are many disorders of the muscle, which include disorders of excitability through mutations in the ion channels (see Chapter 5) as well as inflammation (see Chapter 54) and abnormalities in the structural proteins of the muscle itself. These latter conditions underlie many of the inherited muscular dystrophies of which the best characterized are Duchenne's and the limb girdle muscular dystrophies. *Duchenne's muscular dystrophy (DMD)* is an X-linked disorder in which there is a deletion of the gene coding for the structural protein dystrophin, with the milder form of the disease *(Becker's muscular dystrophy)* having a reduced amount of this same protein. Patients with DMD typically present early in life with clumsiness and difficulty in walking, with an associated wasting of the proximal limb muscles and pseudohypertrophy of the calf muscles. As the disease progresses the patient becomes increasingly disabled, with the development of cardiac and other abnormalities which lead to death, typically in the third decade. Characteristically, these patients have a raised creatine kinase (a marker of muscle damage) as the muscles in these patients are prone to necrosis as a result of the absence of dystrophin. This protein lies beneath the sarcolemma of skeletal (as well as smooth and cardiac) muscle and provides stability and flexibility to the muscle membrane, such that when absent the membrane can be easily disrupted. This allows entry of large quantities of Ca^{2+} which precipitates necrosis by excessive activation of proteases.

The *limb girdle muscular dystrophies (LGMD)*, in contrast, can present at any age with progressive weakness of the proximal limb muscles and a raised creatine kinase. The condition can be inherited in a number of different ways, and recently the autosomal recessive forms of this condition have been found to contain abnormalities in the dystrophin associated glycoproteins, adhalin and the sarcoglycan complex. These proteins link the intracellular dystrophin with components of the extracellular matrix and so are important in maintaining the integrity of the sarcolemma.

11 Skeletal muscle contraction

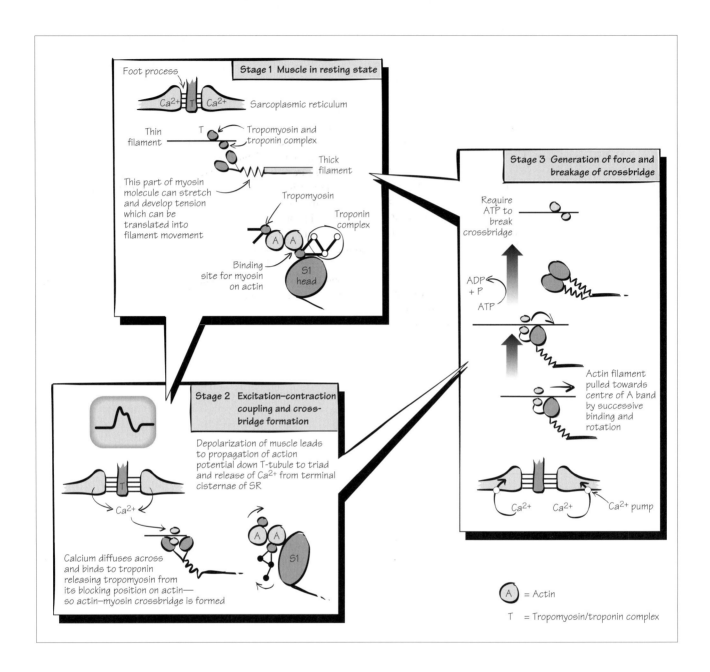

The arrival of the action potential at the neuromuscular junction (NMJ) leads to an influx of Ca^{2+} and the release of vesicles containing acetylcholine (ACh). This binds to the nicotinic ACh receptor (AChR) on the muscle fibre leading to its depolarization and Ca^{2+} release from the sarcoplasmic reticulum (SR) of the muscle. This leads to the removal of the blocking calcium-binding protein complex of **tropomyosin** and **troponin** from **actin**, the main component of the **thin filament**. The removal of this stearic block allows **myosin**, the major component of the **thick filaments**, to bind to actin via a **crossbridge**. The fibres are then pulled past each other; the crossbridge between the two fibres is broken at the end of this power stroke by the **hydrolysis of adenosine triphosphate (ATP)**. The cycle of crossbridge formation and breakage

can then be repeated and the muscle contracts in a ratchet-like fashion. The whole process is termed the **sliding filament hypothesis** of muscle contraction.

The sequence of events in the contraction of muscle is as follows.
• Stage 1: In the resting state the troponin complex holds the tropomyosin in such a position that it blocks myosin from binding to actin (stearic block).
• Stage 2: The arrival of an action potential at the NMJ causes a post-synaptic action potential to be initiated, which is propagated down the specialized invagination of the muscle membrane known as the **transverse tubule (T-tubule)**. This T-tubule conducts the action potential down into the muscle, so that all the muscle fibres can be activated. It

lies adjacent to the terminal cisternae of the SR in a structure known as a **triad**, i.e. a T-tubule lies between two terminal cisternae of the SR (muscle equivalent of smooth endoplasmic reticulum) which contain high concentrations of Ca^{2+}. The T-tubules are linked to the SR by foot processes, which are part of a calcium ion channel. The arrival of the action potential at the triad leads to the release of Ca^{2+} from the terminal cisternae, by a process of mechanical coupling. The action potential opens a common Ca^{2+} ion channel between the T-tubule and SR, which then allows Ca^{2+} to influx down its electrochemical gradient towards the myofibrils.

The Ca^{2+} then binds to the troponin complex and this leads to a rearrangement of the tropomyosin so that the myosin head can now bind to the actin, forming a crosslink or crossbridge.

• Stage 3: Once the myosin has bound to the actin there is a delay before tension develops in the crossbridge. The tension pulls and rotates the actin past the myosin and this causes the muscle to contract. The crossbridge at the end of this power stroke detaches the myosin from actin with hydrolysis of ATP, a process that is also calcium dependent. The whole cycle can then be repeated. The process of crossbridge formation with filament movement is called the **sliding filament hypothesis** of muscle contraction, as the two filaments slide past each other in a ratchet-like fashion as the cycle repeats. The Ca^{2+} released by the terminal cisternae of the SR, allowing the process of crossbridge formation and breakage, is actively taken back up into this structure by a specific Ca^{2+} pump.

Disorders of muscle contraction

Diseases of the muscles, which disrupt their anatomy, will lead to weakness as a consequence of a disorganization of contractile proteins. However, there are some disorders in which there is a disruption of the contractile process itself and examples of this are the rare *periodic paralyses* and *malignant hyperthermia/hyperpyrexia*. In this latter condition there is an abnormality in the ryanodine receptor which is part of the protein complex linking the T-tubule to the SR. This leads, under certain circumstances such as general anaesthesia, to sustained depolarization, contraction and necrosis of muscles resulting in an increase in body temperature and multiorgan dysfunction. In contrast, the periodic paralyses involve abnormalities in the ion channels that can lead to prolonged inexcitability of muscles, which thus become weak and paralysed. These are rare disorders and respiratory muscles are not involved and the paralysis can be provoked by a number of insults such as exercise or high carbohydrate meals.

It is also important to remember that disorders of muscle contraction occur as a consequence of abnormalities at the NMJ (see Chapter 7), as well as with some inborn errors of metabolism. These latter *metabolic myopathies* involve inherited defects in either carbohydrate or lipid metabolism which lead to either episodic exercise-induced symptoms or chronic progressive weakness.

12 The organization of the spinal cord

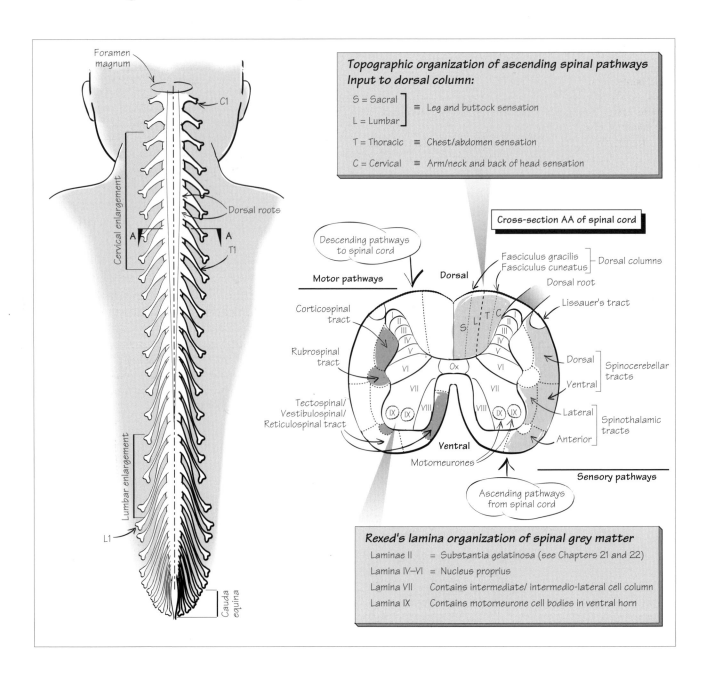

Topographic organization of ascending spinal pathways
Input to dorsal column:

S = Sacral ⎤
⎥ ≡ Leg and buttock sensation
L = Lumbar ⎦

T = Thoracic ≡ Chest/abdomen sensation

C = Cervical ≡ Arm/neck and back of head sensation

Cross-section AA of spinal cord

Rexed's lamina organization of spinal grey matter

Laminae II = Substantia gelatinosa (see Chapters 21 and 22)

Lamina IV–VI = Nucleus proprius

Lamina VII Contains intermediate/ intermedio-lateral cell column

Lamina IX Contains motorneurone cell bodies in ventral horn

Overall structure

The spinal cord lies within the vertebral canal and extends from the foramen magnum to the lower border of the first lumbar vertebra and is enlarged at two sites (cervical and lumbar regions) corresponding to the innervations of the upper and lower limbs (see Chapter 1). The lower part of the vertebral canal (below L1) contains the lower lumbar and sacral nerves and is known as the **cauda equina**.

Sensory nerve fibres enter the spinal cord via the **dorsal (posterior) roots** and their accompanying cell bodies are located in the dorsal root ganglia, while the motor and preganglionic autonomic fibres exit via the **ventral (or anterior) root**, together with some mostly unmyelinated afferent fibres. The **motor cell bodies (or motorneurones)** are found in the ventral horn of the spinal cord, while the preganglionic cell bodies

of the sympathetic nervous system are found in the **intermedio-lateral column** of the spinal cord.

The neuronal cell bodies that make up the central grey matter of the cord are organized into a series of **laminae (of Rexed)**. The white matter surrounding this is composed of myelinated and unmyelinated axons constituting the ascending and descending spinal tracts.

Organization of sensory afferent fibres entering the spinal cord

Sensory information from the peripheral receptors is relayed by primary afferent nerve fibres which terminate in layers I–V of the dorsal horn, the site for termination being different for different receptors. However, in reality, many afferent fibres divide (into an ascending and a descending branch) as they enter the spinal cord so that synaptic contact can be made both with many interneurones in the dorsal horn, as well as up and down the cord through Lissauer's tract.

Sensory processing in the dorsal horn

Typically, a number of primary afferents make synaptic contact with a single dorsal horn neurone. This **convergence** of input has the effect of reducing the acuity (accuracy) of stimulus location. However, the process of **lateral inhibition** helps minimize this loss of acuity by promoting the inhibition of submaximally activated fibre inputs and thus increasing spatial contrast in the sensory input. The dorsal horn receives a number of descending inputs from supraspinal structures that are important in modulating the processing of sensory information through the spinal cord (see, for example, Chapter 22).

Ascending sensory pathways in spinal cord

The spinothalamic tract (STT), also known as the anterolateral system, spinocerebellar and dorsal columns (DCs) are the major ascending pathways of the spinal cord (see Appendix 2). Each tract relays specific information in a topographical fashion, i.e. the sensory information from different parts of the body is conserved in the organization of the ascending pathways. Inputs from the more rostral parts of the body (arm as opposed to leg) supply fibres that lie more laterally in the ascending pathway. Both the DC and STT **decussate** (fibres cross the midline) and therefore the sensory information they relay is ultimately processed in the **contralateral** cerebral hemisphere. However, the site at which this decussation occurs is different for the two pathways, with the anterolateral system crossing the midline in the spinal cord while the DCs decussate in the lower medulla after synapsing in the DC nuclei and forming the medial lemniscus (see Chapters 20 and 21).

Spinal motorneurones

α- and γ-motorneurones (MNs) are both found in the ventral (anterior) horn. The α-MN is one of the largest neurones found in the nervous system and innervates skeletal muscle fibres, while the γ-MN innervates the intrafusal muscle fibres of the muscle spindle (see Chapter 33). The cervical cord MNs innervate the arm muscles while the lumbar and sacral MNs innervate the leg musculature. The MNs are arranged **somatotopically** across the ventral horn such that the more medially placed MNs innervate proximal muscles, while those located more laterally innervate distal muscles (see Chapter 34).

Descending motor tracts

There are a number of descending motor pathways that are defined by their site of origin within the brain (see Appendix 2). The corticospinal (CoST) or pyramidal tract originates in the cerebral cortex and with the rubrospinal tract innervates the laterally placed MNs that supply the distal musculature. In contrast, the remainder of the extrapyramidal tracts (vestibulo-, reticulo- and tectospinal) tracts innervate the more ventromedially placed MNs that control the axial musculature (see Chapters 34–37).

Clinical features of spinal cord damage (see Chapters 31 and 41)

A knowledge of the organizational anatomy of the spinal cord allows one to predict the pattern of deficits with damage, which is of great value in clinical neurology. Examples of specific spinal cord lesions and syndromes illustrating this point are discussed in Chapters 31 and 34.

13 Anatomy of the brainstem

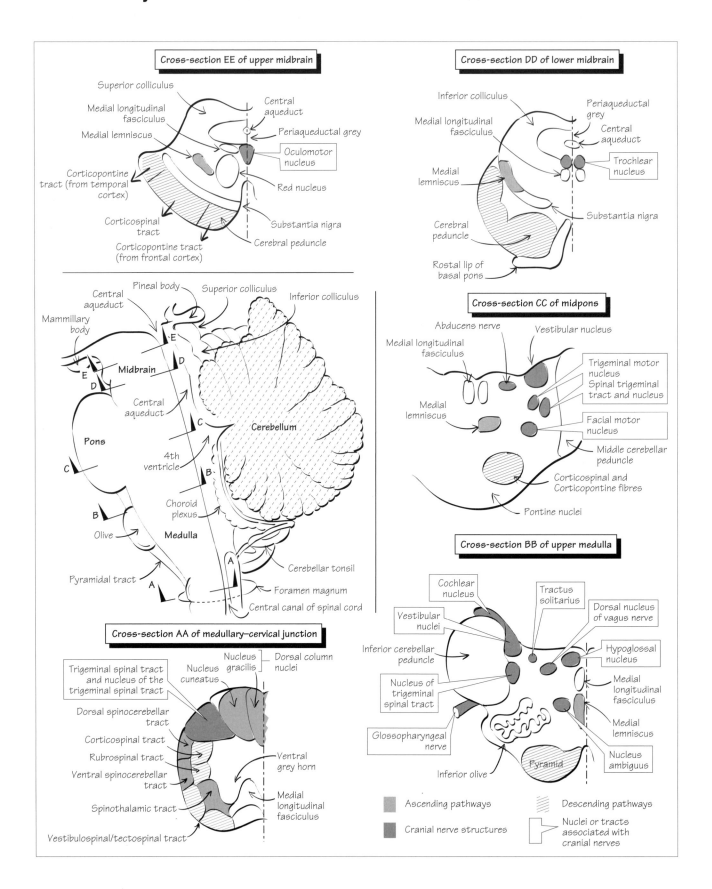

Cross-section EE of upper midbrain

Superior colliculus
Medial longitudinal fasciculus
Medial lemniscus
Corticopontine tract (from temporal cortex)
Corticospinal tract
Corticopontine tract (from frontal cortex)
Central aqueduct
Periaqueductal grey
Oculomotor nucleus
Red nucleus
Substantia nigra
Cerebral peduncle

Cross-section DD of lower midbrain

Inferior colliculus
Medial longitudinal fasciculus
Medial lemniscus
Cerebral peduncle
Rostal lip of basal pons
Periaqueductal grey
Central aqueduct
Trochlear nucleus
Substantia nigra

Central aqueduct
Pineal body
Superior colliculus
Inferior colliculus
Mammillary body
Midbrain
Central aqueduct
Pons
Cerebellum
4th ventricle
Choroid plexus
Olive
Medulla
Pyramidal tract
Cerebellar tonsil
Foramen magnum
Central canal of spinal cord

Cross-section CC of midpons

Abducens nerve
Medial longitudinal fasciculus
Vestibular nucleus
Medial lemniscus
Trigeminal motor nucleus
Spinal trigeminal tract and nucleus
Facial motor nucleus
Middle cerebellar peduncle
Corticospinal and Corticopontine fibres
Pontine nuclei

Cross-section BB of upper medulla

Cochlear nucleus
Vestibular nuclei
Inferior cerebellar peduncle
Nucleus of trigeminal spinal tract
Glossopharyngeal nerve
Inferior olive
Tractus solitarius
Dorsal nucleus of vagus nerve
Hypoglossal nucleus
Medial longitudinal fasciculus
Medial lemniscus
Nucleus ambiguus
Pyramid

Cross-section AA of medullary–cervical junction

Trigeminal spinal tract and nucleus of the trigeminal spinal tract
Dorsal spinocerebellar tract
Corticospinal tract
Rubrospinal tract
Ventral spinocerebellar tract
Spinothalamic tract
Vestibulospinal/tectospinal tract
Nucleus cuneatus
Nucleus gracilis
Dorsal column nuclei
Ventral grey horn
Medial longitudinal fasciculus

Ascending pathways
Cranial nerve structures
Descending pathways
Nuclei or tracts associated with cranial nerves

The brainstem consists of that part of the brain that begins at the **foramen magnum** and extends to the cerebral peduncles and thalamus. It consists of the **medulla, pons** and **midbrain** and is located anterior to the cerebellum to which it is connected by three pairs of cerebellar peduncles. It contains the following.
- The nuclei for 10 of the 12 pairs of **cranial nerves** (see Chapter 14), the exceptions being the olfactory and optic nerves.
- The apparatus for controlling eye movements which includes the third, fourth and sixth cranial nerves (see Chapter 40).
- The monoaminergic nuclei that project widely throughout the CNS (see Chapters 9, 21 and 44).
- Areas that are vital in the control of respiration and the cardiovascular system, as well as the autonomic nervous system (see Chapters 42 and 44).
- Areas important in the control of consciousness, which include some of the monoaminergic nuclei (see Chapter 44).
- A number of ascending and descending pathways linking the spinal cord to supraspinal structures, such as the cerebral cortex and cerebellum, some of which take their origin from the brainstem (see Chapters 12, 18, 20, 21, 32, 34–37).

A number of structures found within the brainstem are worthy of special comment.
- The **dorsal column nuclei** represent the primary site of termination of the fibres conveyed in the dorsal columns (DCs), responsible for light touch, vibration perception and joint position sense. The relay neurones in this structure send axons that decussate in the lower medulla to form the **medial lemniscus** which synapses within the thalamus (see Chapter 20).
- The **pyramid** which represents the descending corticospinal tract (CoST) in the medulla, a pathway that decussates at the lower border of this structure.
- The **tractus solitarius** and **nucleus ambiguus** are associated with taste and the motor innervation of the pharynx by the glossopharyngeal and vagus nerves (see Chapter 14).
- The **inferior olive** in the medulla receives inputs from a number of sources and provides the climbing fibre input to the cerebellum (see Chapters 37 and 47).

- The **cerebellar peduncles** convey information to and from the cerebellum (see Chapter 37).
- The **medial longitudinal fasciculus** originates in the vestibular nucleus and projects rostrally connecting some of the oculomotor nuclei (third and sixth cranial nerves) as well as caudally to form part of the vestibulospinal tract (see Chapter 40).
- The **vestibular nucleus** has important connections from the ear and projects to the spinal cord and cerebellum as well as other brainstem structures (see Chapters 28, 34 and 37).
- The **substantia nigra** in the midbrain contains both dopamine and γ-aminobutyric acid (GABA) neurones, forms part of the basal ganglia and is involved in the control of movement (see Chapters 38–40). The loss of its dopaminergic neurones is the major pathological event in Parkinson's disease (see Chapter 39).
- The **red nucleus** in the midbrain is intimately associated with the cerebellum, and is the site of origin for the rubrospinal tract which, with the CoST, forms the lateral descending pathway of motor control (see Chapters 12, 34–36).
- The **periaqueductal grey matter** of the mesencephalon is an area rich in endogenous opioids and thus is important in the supraspinal modulation of nociception (see Chapter 21).
- The **central aqueduct of Sylvius** running through the midbrain connects the third to the fourth ventricle, and narrowing of it (stenosis) can cause hydrocephalus (see Chapter 16).
- The **cerebral peduncles** contain the descending motor pathways from the cerebral cortex to the spinal cord and brainstem, especially the pons (see Chapter 32).
- The **inferior colliculus** in the midbrain is part of the auditory system (see Chapter 27) while the **superior colliculus** is more involved with visual processing and eye movement control (see Chapters 24 and 40). Thus, damage to the brainstem can have devastating consequences, although small lesions can often be localized with great accuracy because of the number of structures located within this small area of the brain. The most common causes of lesions in this part of the brain are either inflammatory (e.g. *multiple sclerosis*; see Chapter 54) or vascular in nature (see Chapter 17). However, disorders of the brainstem can also be seen with tumours (see Chapter 4) and a host of other conditions.

14 Cranial nerves

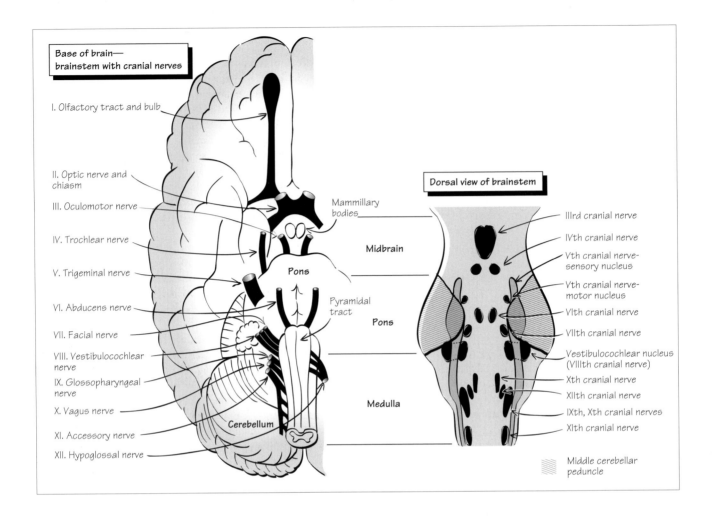

Base of brain— brainstem with cranial nerves

I. Olfactory tract and bulb

II. Optic nerve and chiasm

III. Oculomotor nerve

IV. Trochlear nerve

V. Trigeminal nerve

VI. Abducens nerve

VII. Facial nerve

VIII. Vestibulocochlear nerve

IX. Glossopharyngeal nerve

X. Vagus nerve

XI. Accessory nerve

XII. Hypoglossal nerve

Mammillary bodies

Midbrain

Pons

Pyramidal tract

Pons

Medulla

Cerebellum

Dorsal view of brainstem

IIIrd cranial nerve

IVth cranial nerve

Vth cranial nerve- sensory nucleus

Vth cranial nerve- motor nucleus

VIth cranial nerve

VIIth cranial nerve

Vestibulocochlear nucleus (VIIIth cranial nerve)

Xth cranial nerve

XIIth cranial nerve

IXth, Xth cranial nerves

XIth cranial nerve

Middle cerebellar peduncle

Cranial nerves

I Olfactory nerve

The receptors for olfaction are found within the nasal mucosa, and their axons project through the cribriform plate to the olfactory bulb on the undersurface of the frontal lobe (see Chapter 29). This cranial nerve therefore does not originate or pass through the brainstem, but is a central nervous system (CNS) structure.

II Optic nerve

The photoreceptors in the eye project via ganglion cells to the CNS via the optic nerve. The nerve passes through the optic canal into the brain to form the optic chiasm, whence the fibres pass back as the optic tract to the lateral geniculate nucleus and from there as the optic radiation to the visual cortex (see Chapter 24). This cranial nerve therefore does not originate or pass through the brainstem, although it does have a projection to the midbrain which is important in controlling the **pupillary response to light** (see Chapter 24), as well as to the hypothalamus which helps determine circadian rhythm (see Chapter 43).

III Oculomotor nerve

This originates in the midbrain at the level of the superior colliculus and supplies all the extraocular muscles apart from the lateral rectus which is supplied by the abducens (sixth cranial) nerve and superior oblique which is supplied by the trochlear (fourth cranial) nerve. The oculomotor nerve also carries the parasympathetic innervation to the eye as well as providing the major innervation of levator palpebrae superioris. A complete third nerve palsy causes the eye to lie 'down and out' with a fixed dilated unresponsive pupil and **ptosis** (droopy eyelid). Common causes of this are a posterior communicating artery aneurysm or a microvascular insult to the nerve itself as occurs in diabetes mellitus, for example.

IV Trochlear nerve

This nerve originates in the midbrain at the level of the inferior colliculus, and passes out of the brainstem dorsally. It supplies the superior oblique muscle and damage to this nerve causes double vision (diplopia) on looking down. A common cause of IV nerve palsy is head trauma.

V Fifth cranial or trigeminal nerve

The trigeminal nerve has both a motor and sensory function. The motor nucleus is situated at the midpontine level, medial to the main sensory nucleus of the trigeminal nerve, and receives an input from the motor cortex (see Chapter 35). It supplies the muscles of mastication. Sensation from the whole face (including the cornea) passes to the brainstem in the trigeminal nerve, and synapses in three major nuclear complexes: the nucleus of the spinal tract of the trigeminal nerve; the main sensory nucleus of the trigeminal nerve; and the mesencephalic nucleus. Sensation from the face is relayed via the three branches of the trigeminal nerve: the ophthalmic division that supplies the forehead; the maxillary division that supplies the cheek; and the mandibular branch that supplies the jaw — with the more rostral fibres (ophthalmic branch fibres) passing to the lowest part of the nucleus of the spinal tract in the upper cervical cord. These brainstem trigeminal nuclei in turn project to the thalamus as part of the somatosensory and pain systems (see Chapters 20–22). Damage to the trigeminal nerve results in weak jaw opening and chewing, coupled to facial sensory loss and an absent corneal reflex, and is usually caused by intrinsic lesions of the brainstem or damage to the branches as they pass out of the skull and cavernous sinus.

VI Sixth cranial or abducens nerve

This originates from the dorsal lower portion of the pons and supplies the lateral rectus muscle. Damage to it results in horizontal diplopia when looking to the lesioned side and can be caused by local brainstem pathology or can be a false localizing sign in raised intracranial pressure.

VII Seventh cranial or facial nerve

This is predominantly a motor nerve, although it does carry parasympathetic fibres to the lacrimal and salivary glands (via the greater superficial petrosal nerve and chorda tympani) as well as sensation from the anterior two-thirds of the tongue (via the chorda tympani). The motor nucleus for the facial nerve originates in the pons, and supplies all the muscles of the face except for those involved in mastication.

Damage to this nerve is not uncommon and can occur at any site along its long course, as it passes out of the brainstem through the internal auditory meatus, middle ear and mastoid and through the stylomastoid foramen and into the soft tissue structures of the face. A lesion of this nerve at any of these sites produces a lower facial nerve palsy with weakness of all the facial muscles ipsilateral to the side of the lesion. In addition, there is a loss of taste on the anterior two-thirds of the tongue if the lesion occurs proximal to the departure of the chorda tympani. This is most commonly seen in *Bell's palsy*. In contrast, damage to the descending motor input to the facial nucleus from the cortex (an upper motorneurone facial palsy) causes weakness of the lower part of the contralateral face only, as the musculature of the upper part of the face has an upper motorneurone innervation from the motor cortex of both hemispheres (see Chapters 35, 36 and 41).

VIII Eighth cranial or vestibulocochlear nerve

This conveys information from the cochlea (the auditory or cochlear nerve; see Chapters 26 and 27) as well as the semicircular canals and otolith organs (the vestibular nerve; see Chapter 28). Damage to this nerve (e.g. in *acoustic neuromas*), causes disturbances in balance with deafness and tinnitus (a ringing noise).

IX Ninth cranial or glossopharyngeal nerve

The glossopharyngeal nerve contains motor, sensory and parasympathetic fibres. The motor fibres originate from the rostral nucleus ambiguus and supply the stylopharyngeus muscle, while the sensory fibres synapse in the tractus solitarius (or nucleus of the solitary tract) and provide taste and sensation from the posterior tongue and pharynx. The parasympathetic fibres originate in the inferior salivatory nucleus and provide an input to the parotid gland. Damage to this nerve is usually in conjunction with the vagus nerve (see below) and typically is seen with lesions in the lower brainstem.

X Tenth cranial or vagus nerve

This nerve provides a motor input to the soft palate, pharynx and larynx, which originates in the dorsal motor nucleus of the vagus and nucleus ambiguus. It also has a minor sensory role, conveying taste from the epiglottis and sensation from the pinna, but has a significant parasympathetic role (see Chapter 42). Damage to the vagus nerve causes dysphagia and articulation disturbances and, as with glossopharyngeal nerve lesions, there may be a loss of the gag reflex. This reflex involves tongue retraction and elevation of the pharyngeal musculature in response to a sensory stimulus on the posterior pharynx.

XI Eleventh cranial or spinal accessory nerve

This is purely motor in nature and originates from the nucleus ambiguus in the medulla and the accessory nucleus in the upper cervical spinal cord and supplies the sternocleidomastoid and trapezius muscles. Damage to it causes weakness in these muscles, although in practice this nerve is usually damaged in conjunction with other lower cranial nerves.

XII Twelfth cranial or hypoglossal nerve

The hypoglossal nerve provides the motor innervation of the tongue. Its fibres originate from the hypoglossal nucleus in the posterior part of the medulla. Damage to this nerve causes wasting and weakness in the tongue which leads to problems of swallowing and speech, and is most commonly seen in *motorneurone disease* (see Chapter 52). Isolated damage of this nerve is rare and it is more commonly affected with other lower cranial nerves (e.g. IX, X, XI cranial nerves) and in such cases the patient may present with a *bulbar palsy*. A *pseudobulbar palsy*, in contrast, refers to a loss of the descending cortical input to these cranial nerve nuclei.

15 The organization of the cerebral cortex

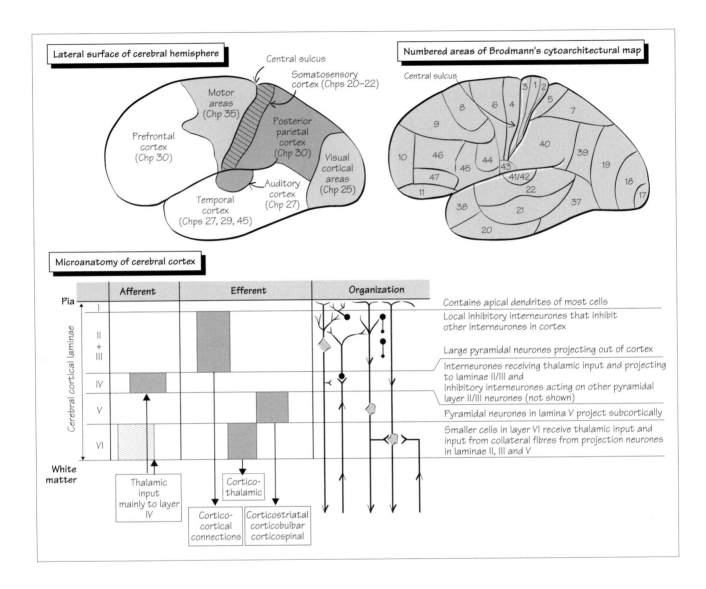

The organization of the outer layer of the cerebral hemisphere or **cerebral cortex** (neocortex) can be considered in various ways. Some of the earliest ways of doing this with cytoarchitectural maps are still used (e.g. **Brodmann's map** of the human brain from 1909). This way of mapping the cortex equates to some extent with the functional organization of this structure into motor, sensory and association areas, as evidenced by the **laminar organization** of the cortex. An area of cortex that is predominantly sensory in character has a prominent layer IV within it as this is the site of termination for thalamic afferent fibres, while cortical motor areas have a prominent layer V. An alternative approach is to view the cortex as being organized vertically. This vertical organization has become known as the **columnar hypothesis** and proposes that the 'column' of cortex is the basic unit of cortical processing and that the phylogenetic development of the cortex has involved an increase in the number of these columns. This explains why the enlargement of the neocortex in primates has been accomplished by

a great expansion of its surface area, without striking changes in the number of neurones in a vertical penetration across the thickness of the cortex.

Anatomical organization of the cerebral cortex

The neocortex is classically described as consisting of six layers, although in certain areas of the cerebral cortex further subdivisions are used, e.g. the primary visual cortex (see Chapter 25). The thalamic afferent fibres, relaying sensory information, project to layer IV often with a smaller input to layer VI, and terminate in discrete patches thus ensuring that sensory information from a specific location and/or receptor type is relayed to a specific area of cortex. This input then synapses on interneurones within the cortex which in turn project vertically to neurones in layers II, III and V, which in turn project to other cortical and subcortical sites, respectively. Thus, the weight of synaptic relations within the cerebral cortex is in the vertical direction, although corticocortical connections linking columns of similar characteristics are found. This arrangement of synaptic connections is well seen in the somatosensory and visual cortices (see Chapters 20 and 25), and it means that a given sensory input from the thalamus will be analysed by a vertical column of cortical neurones. In cortical areas with a motor function, the motor output from that cortical area is such that it is directed back at the motorneurones (MNs) controlling the muscles that move the sensory receptors which ultimately project to that same area of cortex — so-called input–output coupling (see Chapter 36 for more details).

The anatomical evidence thus supports the notion of a vertical columnar organization to the neocortex, but further evidence comes from developmental and neurophysiological studies.

Developmental organization of the cerebral cortex

In the mammalian central nervous system (CNS) the entire population of cortical neurones is produced by a process of migration from the proliferative zones that are situated around the cavities of the cerebral ventricles. The **radial glial fibres** which guide and may even give rise to the migrating neurones span the fetal cerebral wall and direct the neurones to their correct cortical location in the developing **cortical plate** from the **ventricular and subventricular zones** (see Chapter 2). Thus, developmentally, the cortex forms in a vertical fashion.

Neurophysiological organization of the cerebral cortex

Neurophysiologically, if a recording electrode is passed at right angles through the cortex, it encounters cells with similar properties. However, if the electrode is passed tangentially then cells shift their response characteristics. This has been shown in all the primary sensory cortices, as well as the primary motor cortex (see Chapters 20, 25 and 36).

This columnar organization of the cortex means that topography can be maintained and that the reorganization of the cortex in the event of a change in the peripheral input is relatively straightforward (see Chapter 47).

Functional organization of the cerebral cortex

The relationship of cortical columns to one another raises many inter-esting questions as to the mode of function employed by the cerebral cortex. The original models on information processing in the cortex proposed that it was performed in a serial fashion, such that the cortical cells form a series of levels in a **hierarchy**. Thus, one set of cells perform a relatively straightforward analysis which then converges on another population of neurones that perform a more complex analysis (see, for example, Chapter 25). The ultimate prediction of these hierarchical models is that one neurone at the top of the hierarchy will register the percept—the **'grandmother' cell**. However, the discovery of the X, Y and W classes of ganglion cells in the retina (see Chapter 23) led to the development of a competing theory that proposed that information is analysed by a series of **parallel pathways**, with each pathway analysing one specific aspect of the sensory stimulus (e.g. colour or motion with visual stimuli; see Chapter 25). This theory does not exclude hierarchical processing but relegates it to the mode of analysis within separate parallel pathways. In practice, however, the cortex employs both modes of analysis.

It should be stressed that cortical columns are not to be viewed as a static mosaic structure, as one column may be a member of a number of different pathways of analysis. This organization has been termed the **distributed system theory** and describes the brain as a complex of widely and reciprocally interconnected systems, with the dynamic interplay of neural activity within and between these systems as the very essence of brain function. Consequently, one column may be a member of many distributed systems, because each distributed system is specific for one feature of a stimulus and one column may code for several features of the stimulus. An analogy for viewing this is to imagine the London underground system where each station is defined by the connections it has with other stations. Thus, one station may be part of many different lines and providing to each a unique quality. This analogy also helps explain the plasticity within the CNS, as damage to a station can be compensated for, up to a point, by the remaining networks as there is a degree of redundancy to the representation. However, if there is severe damage, especially of important centres or the peripheral terminals, then the system cannot compensate and lasting deficits ensue.

16 Meninges and cerebrospinal fluid

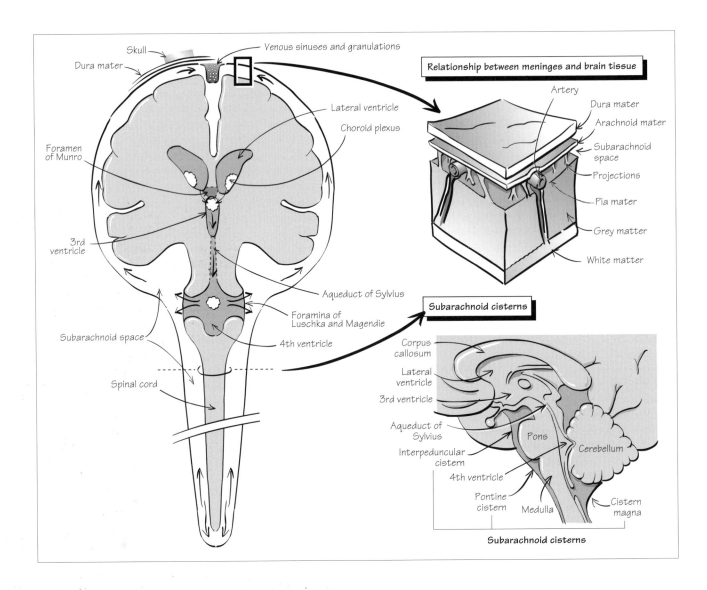

Within the skull the brain is enclosed by three protective layers which also extend down the spinal cord. The **dura mater** is a thick tough membrane lying close to the skull and vertebrae and innervated by afferent fibres of the trigeminal nerve and upper cervical nerves. Headache can be associated with disturbance or inflammation of the dura. Adjacent to this is the **arachnoid mater**, a thin membrane with thread-like processes that project into the subarachnoid space and make contact with the delicate **pia mater** which envelopes the spinal cord and contours of the brain surface and dips into the sulci.

The **subarachnoid space** is filled with cerebrospinal fluid (CSF) and also accommodates major arteries, branches of which project down through the pia into the central nervous system (CNS). At specific sites the size of the subarachnoid space increases to form **cisterns**. These are particularly prevalent in the region of the brainstem and the largest is the **cisterna magna** found between the cerebellum and medulla.

The meninges extend caudally enclosing the spinal cord. Here the dura is attached to the foramen magnum at its upper limit and projects down to the second sacral vertebra.

Cerebrospinal fluid production and circulation

CSF is secreted by the **choroid plexuses** which are found primarily in the ventricles. The rate of production varies between about 300 and 500 mL/24 h and the ventricular volume is about 75 mL. CSF is similar to blood plasma although it contains less albumin and glucose. After production, CSF flows from the lateral ventricles into the third ventricle via the intraventricular foramina of Munro and then passes into the fourth ventricle via the central aqueduct of Sylvius and into the subarachnoid space via the foramina of Luschka and Magendie. From the subarachnoid space at the base of the brain CSF flows rostrally over the cerebral hemispheres or down into the spinal cord.

CSF reabsorption occurs within the superior sagittal and related venous sinuses. Arachnoid **granulations** are minute pouches of the arachnoid membrane projecting through the dura into the venous sinuses. The exact mechanism by which CSF is reabsorbed is not clear but does involve the movement of all CSF constituents into the venous blood.

As well as playing an important part in maintaining a constant intracerebral chemical environment (see below), the CSF also helps to protect the brain from mechanical damage by reducing the effect of impact damage experienced by the head.

Blood–brain barrier

The blood–brain barrier (BBB) used to be thought of as a single physical barrier preventing the passage of molecules and cells into the brain. More recently, however, it has been shown to be made up of a series of different transport systems for facilitating or restricting the movement of molecules across the blood–CSF interface. A characteristic of cerebral capillary endothelial cells is the presence of tight junctions between such cells, which are induced and maintained by astrocytic foot processes (see Chapter 4). These unusually tight junctions reduce opportunities for the movement of large molecules and cells, and thus require the existence of specific transport systems for the passage of certain critical molecules into the brain.

Small molecules such as glucose pass readily into the CSF despite not being lipid soluble. Larger protein molecules do not enter the brain but there are a number of carrier mechanisms that enable the transport of other sugars and some amino acids to occur. The effect of the barrier is to maintain a constant intracerebral chemical environment and protect against osmotic challenges, while granting the CNS relative immunological privilege by preventing cells from entering (see Chapter 54). However, from a therapeutic point of view the barrier reduces or prevents the delivery of many drugs (e.g. antibiotics) into the brain.

Clinical disorders

Hydrocephalus is defined as dilatation of the ventricular system and so can be seen in cases of cerebral atrophy, e.g. dementia (compensatory hydrocephalus). However, hydrocephalus can also occur as a result of increased pressure within the ventricular system, secondary to an obstruction in the flow of CSF (obstructive hydrocephalus). This typically occurs at the outlets from the fourth ventricle into the subarachnoid space, where the obstruction may be linked to the presence of a tumour, congenital malformation or the sequelae of a previous infection (see below). Alternatively, the flow of CSF from the third to the fourth ventricle may be impaired as a result of the development of **central aqueduct stenosis**. Hydrocephalus is also seen in conditions of oversecretion of CSF (e.g. tumours of the choroid plexus) as well as reduced absorption as occurs in **spina bifida**.

The symptomatology of hydrocephalus is varied but classically the patient presents with features of raised intracranial pressure (early morning headache, nausea, vomiting) and, in acute rises of pressure, altered levels of consciousness with brief periods of visual loss. Overall, probably the most common cause of raised intracranial pressure is a glial tumour (see Chapter 4) producing an effect by virtue of its mass, although such tumours in the posterior fossa can also directly cause hydrocephalus which may contribute to the raised intracranial pressure.

In obstructive hydrocephalus the treatment focuses on draining excess CSF using a variety of shunts linking the ventricles to either the heart (atrium) or the peritoneal cavity.

Meningitis

Meningitis or inflammation within the meningeal membrane can be caused by a number of different organisms. In acute infection there is the rapid spread of inflammation throughout the entire subarachnoid space of the brain and spinal cord, which produces the symptoms of headache, pyrexia, vomiting, neck stiffness (meningism) and, in severe forms of the disease, reduced levels of consciousness. The early administration of antibiotics is essential although the need to use and the type of antibiotic employed will depend on the nature of the organism responsible for the inflammation.

In other cases the infection or inflammation may follow a more subacute course, such as tuberculous meningitis or sarcoidosis. In cases such as this, secondary hydrocephalus may ensue as a result of meningeal thickening at the base of the brain obstructing CSF flow.

Rarely, tumours can spread up the meninges giving a **malignant meningitis**. This characteristically presents as an evolving cranial nerve or nerve root syndrome with pain. This is to be distinguished from primary tumours of the meninges—**meningiomas**—which are slow growing and benign and typically present with epileptic seizures or deficits secondary to compression of neighbouring CNS structures.

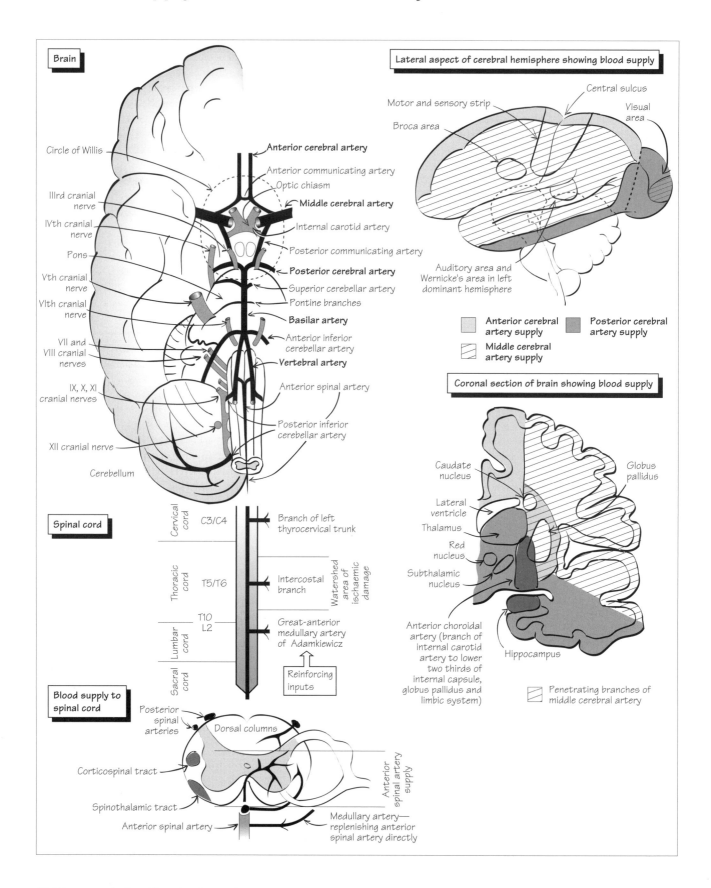

Brain

Circle of Willis

IIIrd cranial nerve

IVth cranial nerve

Pons

Vth cranial nerve

VIth cranial nerve

VII and VIII cranial nerves

IX, X, XI cranial nerves

XII cranial nerve

Cerebellum

Anterior cerebral artery

Anterior communicating artery

Optic chiasm

Middle cerebral artery

Internal carotid artery

Posterior communicating artery

Posterior cerebral artery

Superior cerebellar artery

Pontine branches

Basilar artery

Anterior inferior cerebellar artery

Vertebral artery

Anterior spinal artery

Posterior inferior cerebellar artery

Lateral aspect of cerebral hemisphere showing blood supply

Central sulcus

Motor and sensory strip

Visual area

Broca area

Auditory area and Wernicke's area in left dominant hemisphere

Anterior cerebral artery supply

Posterior cerebral artery supply

Middle cerebral artery supply

Coronal section of brain showing blood supply

Caudate nucleus

Globus pallidus

Lateral ventricle

Thalamus

Red nucleus

Subthalamic nucleus

Anterior choroidal artery (branch of internal carotid artery to lower two thirds of internal capsule, globus pallidus and limbic system)

Hippocampus

Penetrating branches of middle cerebral artery

Spinal cord

Cervical cord — C3/C4

Thoracic cord — T5/T6

Lumbar cord — T10 L2

Sacral cord

Branch of left thyrocervical trunk

Intercostal branch

Watershed area of ischaemic damage

Great-anterior medullary artery of Adamkiewicz

Reinforcing inputs

Blood supply to spinal cord

Posterior spinal arteries

Dorsal columns

Corticospinal tract

Spinothalamic tract

Anterior spinal artery

Anterior spinal artery supply

Medullary artery— replenishing anterior spinal artery directly

Blood supply to the brain

The arterial blood supply to the brain comes from four vessels: the right and left internal carotid and vertebral arteries. The **vertebral arteries** enter the skull through the foramen magnum and unite to supply blood to the brainstem (**basilar artery**) and posterior parts of the cerebral hemisphere (**posterior cerebral arteries**)—the whole network constituting the posterior circulation. The **internal carotid arteries (ICAs)** traverse the skull in the carotid canal and the cavernous sinus before piercing the dura and entering the middle cranial fossa just lateral to the optic chiasm. They then divide and supply blood to the anterior and middle parts of the cerebral hemispheres (**anterior and middle cerebral arteries; ACAs and MCAs, respectively**). In addition, the posterior and anterior cerebral circulations anastomose at the base of the brain in the **circle of Willis**, with the anterior and posterior communicating arteries offering the potential to maintain cerebral circulation in the event of a major arterial occlusion. Such a situation is not uncommonly seen in atherosclerotic disease where a slowly progressive stenosis of the ICA allows the collateral system to develop prior to the final occlusion of the vessel. These patients remain asymptomatic or may experience transient neurological disturbances as microthrombi are thrown off from the stenosing vessel (*transient ischaemic attacks or TIAs*) which stop without a significant deficit once the vessel is completely occluded.

The ICA prior to its terminal bifurcation supplies branches to the pituitary (hypophysial arteries), the eye (ophthalmic artery), parts of the basal ganglia (globus pallidus) and limbic system (anterior choroidal artery) as well as providing the posterior communicating artery. The MCA forms one of the two terminal branches of the ICA and supplies the sensorimotor strip surrounding the central sulcus (with the exception of its medial extension which is supplied by the ACA) as well as the auditory and language cortical areas in the dominant (usually left) hemisphere. Therefore, occlusion of the MCA causes a contralateral paralysis that affects the arm and the lower part of the face and arm especially, with contralateral sensory loss or inattention and a loss of language if the dominant hemisphere is involved (see Chapters 20, 27, 30 and 36). In addition, there are a number of small penetrating branches of the MCA that supply subcortical structures such as the basal ganglia and internal capsule (see below).

The two **ACAs**, which form the other major terminal vessel of the ICA, are connected via the anterior communicating artery and supply blood to the medial portions of the frontal and parietal lobes as well as the corpus callosum. There is an inconstant branch of the ACA, the recurrent artery of Heubner, which supplies part of the basal ganglia (neostriatum) and descending motor pathways in the internal capsule. Occlusion of the ACA characteristically gives paresis of the contralateral leg with sensory loss, and on occasions deficits in gait and micturition with mental impairment and *dyspraxia* (see Chapters 20, 30 and 35).

The **vertebral arteries**, which arise from the subclavian artery, ascend to the brainstem via foramina in the transverse processes of the upper cervical vertebrae. At the level of the lower part of the pons the vertebral arteries unite to form the basilar artery which then ascends before dividing into the two **posterior cerebral arteries (PCAs)** at the superior border of the pons. Each vertebral artery *en route* to forming the basilar artery has a number of branches including the posterior spinal artery, the posterior inferior cerebellar artery (PICA) and the anterior spinal artery. These spinal arteries supply the upper cervical cord (see below), whereas the PICA supplies the lateral part of the medulla and cerebellum. Occlusion of this vessel gives rise to the *lateral medullary syndrome of Wallenberg*.

The **basilar artery** has a number of branches: the anterior inferior cerebellar artery (AICA); the artery to the labyrinth; pontine branches; and the superior cerebellar artery. Occlusion of these branches gives a characteristic clinical picture that can be predicted from the anatomy of the brainstem (see Chapter 13).

The **PCAs** supply blood to the posterior parietal cortex, the occipital lobe and inferior parts of the temporal lobe. Occlusion of these vessels causes a visual field defect (usually a homonymous hemianopia with macular sparing, as this cortical area receives some supply from the MCA; see Chapter 24), amnesic syndromes (see Chapter 45), disorders of language (see Chapter 27) and, occasionally, complex visual perceptual abnormalities (see Chapter 25). The PCA has a number of central perforating or penetrating branches which supply the midbrain, thalamus, subthalamus, posterior internal capsule, optic radiation and cerebral peduncle. Occlusion of these vessels produces midbrain syndromes with a combination of cranial nerve palsies and motor abnormalities; in the case of thalamic involvement, they may also produce a syndrome of pain and dysaesthesia that is hard to treat (see Chapter 22). The small perforating arteries that arise from both the PCA and MCA are commonly affected in hypertension when their occlusion produces small **lacunar infarcts**.

Apart from occlusion, **haemorrhage** from cerebral vessels can occur which may be into the brain substance (intracerebral), the subarachnoid space or both. Such haemorrhages usually occur either in the context of trauma, hypertension or rupture of congenital aneurysms on the circle of Willis (*berry aneurysms*).

Venous drainage of the brain

Venous drainage of the brainstem and cerebellum is directly into the dural venous sinuses adjacent to the posterior cranial fossa. The cerebral hemispheres in contrast have internal and external veins—the external cerebral veins drain the cortex and empty into the superior sagittal sinus (see Chapter 16). This sinus drains into the transverse sinus, then the lateral sinus, before emptying into the internal jugular vein. The internal cerebral veins drain the deep structures of the cerebral hemisphere to the great vein of Galen and thence into the straight sinus. Occlusion of either of these venous systems can occur, causing raised intracranial pressure with or without focal deficits.

Blood supply to the spinal cord

The **blood supply to the spinal cord** comes in the form of a single anterior spinal artery and paired posterior spinal arteries. The anterior spinal artery arises from the vertebral arteries and extends from the level of the lower brainstem to the tip of the conus medullaris. It supplies the ventral surface of the medulla and the anterior two-thirds of the spinal cord. The posterior spinal arteries supply the dorsal third of the spinal cord, and also take their origin from the vertebral arteries. At certain sites along the spinal cord there are a number of reinforcing inputs from other arteries (see figure).

Vascular insults to the spinal cord occur most commonly at the watershed areas in the cord, namely the lower cervical and lower thoracic cord. Occlusion of the anterior spinal artery produces a loss of power and spinothalamic sensory deficit with preservation of the dorsal column sensory modalities (joint position sense and vibration perception; see Chapter 31). Posterior spinal artery occlusions are rare and produce a loss of dorsal column sensory modalities.

18 Sensory systems: an overview

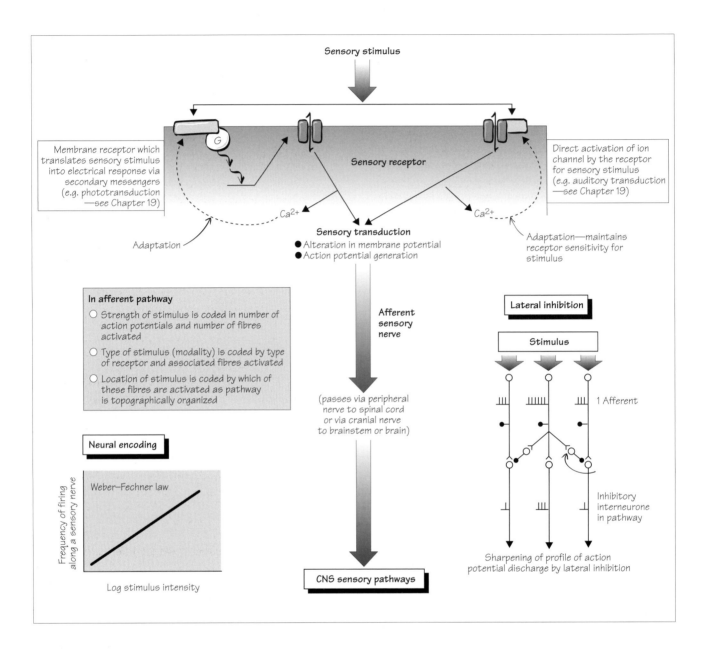

A sensory system is one in which information is conveyed to the spinal cord and brain from peripheral sensory receptors, which in themselves are either specialized neurones or nerve endings. The specialized **sensory receptor**, **afferent axon** and **cell body** together with the synaptic contacts in the spinal cord, are known as the **primary afferent**, and the process by which stimuli from the external environment are converted into electrical signals for transmission through the nervous system is known as **sensory transduction** (see Chapter 19). The signal produced by the sensory receptor is relayed to the central nervous system (CNS) via peripheral or cranial nerves and through a series of synapses eventually projects to a given area of cortex that is then capable of detailed analysis of that sensory input.

There are five main sensory systems in the mammalian nervous system: (i) touch/pressure, proprioception, temperature and pain or the somatosensory system (see Chapters 20–22); (ii) vision (see Chapters 23–25); (iii) hearing and balance (see Chapters 26–28); (iv) taste (see Chapter 29); and (v) smell or olfaction (see Chapter 29). All but the somatosensory pathways are regarded as 'special' senses.

Sensory receptors

Sensory receptors transduce the sensory stimulus either by a process of **direct ion channel activation** (e.g. the auditory system) or **indirectly via a secondary intracellular messenger network** (e.g. the visual system). In both cases the sensory stimulus is converted into an electrical signal that can then be relayed to the CNS either in the form of graded depolarizations/hyperpolarizations leading on to action potentials (e.g. visual system) or the direct generation of action potentials at the level of the receptor (e.g. auditory system; see Chapter 19).

The **specificity or modality** of a sensory system relies on the activation of specialized nerve cells or fibres which are highly specific for different forms of afferent stimuli, e.g. receptors in the retina are highly specific for photons although they may be activated by other stimuli in non-physiological circumstances such as pressure with compression of the eye. The receptor will only respond to stimuli when they are applied within a given region around it (its **receptive field**); an area of skin in the somatosensory system or a part of the retina in the case of photoreceptors, for example. This area or receptive field from which the receptor can be activated is recognized by the CNS as corresponding to a specific site or position in the body or outside world. However, the receptor will only transmit electrical information to the CNS when it receives a stimulus of sufficient intensity to reach the firing **threshold**. The incremental response to a change in stimulus intensity by the receptor gives the receptor its **sensitivity**. Many receptors have a high sensitivity to both the absolute level of stimulus detection and to changes in stimulus intensity because they are capable of both amplifying the original signal by the use of secondary messenger systems, and **adapting** to the presence of a continuous unchanging stimulus (see below and Chapter 19). Some receptors can change their sensitivity by altering the time and area over which they integrate incident stimuli, e.g. retinal rod photoreceptors in darkness. However, with very sensitive receptors the intrinsic instability of the transduction process is termed the **noise** and the challenge for the nervous system is to detect a sensory stimulus response or signal over this background noise (termed the **signal to noise ratio**).

The strength of a sensory stimulus can be coded for at the level of the receptor and its first synapse either in the form of action potentials or graded membrane potentials within the receptor which are subsequently converted into action potentials (see Chapter 19). The **afferent sensory nerve** can code (amongst other things) for the strength of the stimulus, first by increasing the number of afferent fibres activated **(recruitment or spatial coding)** and, secondly, by increasing the number of action potentials generated in each axon per unit time **(temporal or frequency coding)**. However, the relationship between the stimulus strength and the number of action potentials generated is often non-linear because of the limited number of action potentials an axon can conduct by virtue of its refractory period (see Chapter 6).

The receptor, while being able to detect and code for the intensity of a specific sensory stimulus at a specific site, must also be capable of adapting so that it can respond to changes in the sensory information it receives. **Adaptation** is therefore defined as the decrease in receptor sensitivity that occurs in the presence of a maintained stimulus, and intracellular Ca^{2+} is an important mediator of this process in most sensory systems (see Chapter 19). If such a mechanism did not exist then a continuously applied stimulus would greatly reduce the sensitivity or even inactivate the receptor to any other new sensory inputs (e.g. the muscle spindle; see Chapter 33).

Sensory pathways

The coded information from the sensory receptors is relayed to the CNS via peripheral and cranial nerves, with each receptor having an associated axon. Each modality is associated with specific nerves or pathways, e.g. visual information is relayed via the optic nerve (see Chapter 24) while the somatosensory system relays information from a large number of peripheral nerves as well as the trigeminal nerve via the dorsal column–medial lemniscal system and spinothalamic tracts. Thus, each sensory pathway has its own unique input to the CNS, although ultimately most sensory pathways provide an input to the thalamus—the site of that projection being different for each sensory system. This in turn projects to the cortex, although the olfactory pathway primarily projects to limbic structures (see Chapter 29) and the muscle spindle to the cerebellum (see Chapter 37).

Each sensory system has its own area of cortex that is primarily concerned with analysing the sensory information and this area of cortex—the **primary sensory area**—is connected to adjacent cortical areas that perform more complex sensory processing **(secondary sensory areas)**. This in turn projects into the **association areas** (posterior parietal, prefrontal and temporal cortices; see Chapter 30) which then project to the motor and limbic systems (see Chapters 32 and 45). These latter areas are more involved in the processing of sensory information as a cue for moving and generating complex behavioural responses.

The primary sensory cortical areas not only project to secondary sensory areas but also subcortically to their thalamic (and/or brainstem) projecting nuclei. This may be important in augmenting the detection of significant ascending sensory signals. This augmentation probably involves at least two major processes: **lateral inhibition** and **feature detection**. Lateral inhibition is a process by which those cells and axons with the greatest activity are highlighted by the inhibition of adjacent less active ones, which produces greater contrast in the afferent information. Feature detection, on the other hand, corresponds to the selective detection of given features of a sensory stimulus, which can occur at any level from the receptor to the cortex. Ultimately, the perception of any sensory stimulus relies on the synchronous activity of several areas of cerebral cortex (see Chapter 15).

Clinical disorders of the sensory pathways (see Chapter 31)

Damage at different sites in a sensory pathway produces a deficit, the extent and nature of which is dependent on the anatomical location. In general, the most devastating sensory losses are associated with damage to the receptors and their afferent pathways, while supraspinal lesions are often associated with more subtle deficits, which can be 'positive' in nature, e.g. paraesthesiae with focal *epilepsy* originating from the primary sensory cortex, or flashing lights with ischaemia of the visual cortex in *migraine*.

19 Sensory transduction

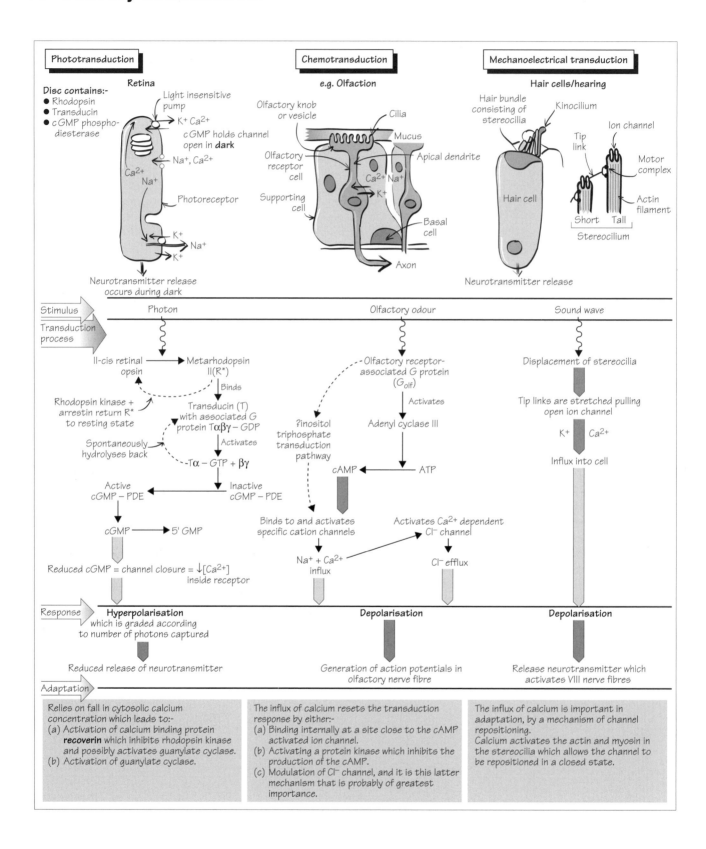

Phototransduction

Retina

Disc contains:-
● Rhodopsin
● Transducin
● cGMP phospho-
diesterase

Light insensitive pump

K⁺ Ca²⁺

cGMP holds channel open in **dark**

Na⁺, Ca²⁺

Ca²⁺
Na⁺

Photoreceptor

K⁺ Na⁺
K⁺

Neurotransmitter release occurs during dark

Chemotransduction

e.g. Olfaction

Olfactory knob or vesicle

Cilia

Mucus

Olfactory receptor cell

Apical dendrite

Ca²⁺ Na⁺

K⁺

Supporting cell

Basal cell

Axon

Mechanoelectrical transduction

Hair cells/hearing

Hair bundle consisting of stereocilia

Kinocilium

Tip link

Ion channel

Motor complex

Hair cell

Actin filament

Short Tall

Stereocilium

Neurotransmitter release

Stimulus → Photon ⟿ | Olfactory odour ⟿ | Sound wave ⟿

Transduction process →

Phototransduction pathway:

11-cis retinal opsin → Metarhodopsin II (R*)

| Binds

Rhodopsin kinase + arrestin return R* to resting state

Transducin (T) with associated G protein Tαβγ – GDP

Spontaneously hydrolyses back

| Activates

-Tα – GTP + βγ

Active cGMP – PDE ← Inactive cGMP – PDE

cGMP → 5' GMP

Reduced cGMP = channel closure = ↓[Ca²⁺] inside receptor

Chemotransduction pathway:

-Olfactory receptor-associated G protein (G_olf)

| Activates

Adenyl cyclase III

?inositol triphosphate transduction pathway

cAMP ← ATP

Binds to and activates specific cation channels

Na⁺ + Ca²⁺ influx

Activates Ca²⁺ dependent Cl⁻ channel

Cl⁻ efflux

Mechanoelectrical pathway:

Displacement of stereocilia

Tip links are stretched pulling open ion channel

K⁺ Ca²⁺

Influx into cell

Response →

Hyperpolarisation which is graded according to number of photons captured

Reduced release of neurotransmitter

Depolarisation

Generation of action potentials in olfactory nerve fibre

Depolarisation

Release neurotransmitter which activates VIII nerve fibres

Adaptation →

Relies on fall in cytosolic calcium concentration which leads to:-
(a) Activation of calcium binding protein **recoverin** which inhibits rhodopsin kinase and possibly activates guanylate cyclase.
(b) Activation of guanylate cyclase.

The influx of calcium resets the transduction response by either:-
(a) Binding internally at a site close to the cAMP activated ion channel.
(b) Activating a protein kinase which inhibits the production of the cAMP.
(c) Modulation of Cl⁻ channel, and it is this latter mechanism that is probably of greatest importance.

The influx of calcium is important in adaptation, by a mechanism of channel repositioning.
Calcium activates the actin and myosin in the stereocilia which allows the channel to be repositioned in a closed state.

Sensory transduction involves the conversion of a stimulus from the external or internal environment into an electrical signal for transmission through the nervous system. This process is performed by all sensory systems and in general involves either a **chemical process** as occurs in the retina, tongue or olfactory epithelium, or a **mechanical process** as occurs in the cochlea and somatosensory systems. These contrasting modes of transduction are best characterized in some of the special senses.

Phototransduction

Phototransduction is the process by which light energy in the form of photons is translated into electrical energy in the form of potential changes in the photoreceptors (rods and cones) in the retina.

Photons are captured in pigments in the photoreceptor outer segment, which results in an amplification process using cyclic guanosine monophosphate (cGMP) as the secondary messenger. This results in reduced cGMP concentrations which leads to channel closure. The closure of these channels, which allow Na^+ and Ca^{2+} to enter the photoreceptor in the dark, leads to a hyperpolarization response, the degree of which is graded according to the number of photons captured by the photoreceptor pigment. The hyperpolarization response leads to reduced glutamate release by the photoreceptor on to bipolar and horizontal cells (see Chapter 23).

The termination of the photoreceptor response to light is multifactorial, but changes in intracellular Ca^{2+} concentration are important. The light insensitive Ca^{2+} pump in the outer segment coupled to the closure of the cation channel leads to a significant reduction in intracellular Ca^{2+} concentrations which is important in terminating the photoreceptor response as well as mediating light (or background) adaptation.

A number of rare congenital forms of **night blindness** have now been associated with specific deficits within the phototransduction pathway.

Olfactory transduction

Olfactory transduction is similarly a chemically mediated process. The olfactory receptor cells are bipolar neurones consisting of a dendrite with a dendritic knob on which are found the cilia, and an axonal part that projects as the olfactory nerve to the olfactory bulb on the underside of the frontal lobe. The presence of cilia, which contain the olfactory receptors, greatly increase the surface area of the olfactory neuroepithelium and so increase the probability of trapping odourant molecules. The binding of the odourant molecule to the receptor leads to the activation of G_{olf} which activates adenylate cyclase type III which hydrolyses adenosine triphosphate (ATP) to cyclic adenosine monophosphate (cAMP). cAMP then binds to and activates specific cation channels, thus allowing Na^+ and Ca^{2+} to influx down their con-

centration gradients. This not only partly depolarizes the receptor, but also leads to the activation of a Ca^{2+}-dependent Cl^- channel and the subsequent Cl^- efflux then further depolarizes the olfactory receptor. There are probably additional transduction processes present in the olfactory receptor using inositol triphosphate as the secondary messenger. This can lead to the generation of action potentials at the cell body which are then conducted down the olfactory nerve axons to the olfactory bulb.

The Ca^{2+} influx is also important in adaptation by resetting the transduction response.

Auditory transduction

In contrast to both phototransduction and olfactory transduction, the process of **auditory transduction** in the inner ear involves the mechanical displacement of stereocilia on the hair cells of the cochlea (see Chapter 26).

The sensory stimulus, a sound wave, causes displacement of the stapedial foot process in the oval window which generates waves in the perilymphatic filled scala vestibuli and tympani of the cochlea. This leads to displacement of the basilar membrane on which the hair cells are to be found in the organ of Corti. These cells transduce the sound waves into an electrical response by a process of mechanotransduction. The stereocilia at the apical end of the hair cell are linked at their tips by tip links, which are attached to ion channels.

The sound causes the stereocilia to be displaced in the direction of the largest stereocilia (or kinocilium) which creates tension within the tip links which then pull open an ion channel. This ion channel then allows K^+ (not Na^+, as the endolymph within the scala media is rich in K^+ and low in Na^+) and Ca^{2+} to flow into the hair cell and by so doing depolarize it. This depolarization leads to the release of neurotransmitter at the base of the hair cell which activates the afferent fibres of the cochlear nerve.

The continued displacement of the stereocilia in response to a sound is countered by a process of adaptation with a repositioning of the ion channel such that it is now shut in response to that degree of tip link tension. This is achieved by the influx of Ca^{2+} through the ion transduction channels.

A number of syndromes with congenital deafness have now been identified as being caused by abnormalities in the myosin found in hair cells.

Other transduction processes

Transduction in the somatosensory receptors, nociceptors, thermoreceptors, taste receptors and muscle spindle are discussed in Chapters 20, 21, 29 and 33, respectively.

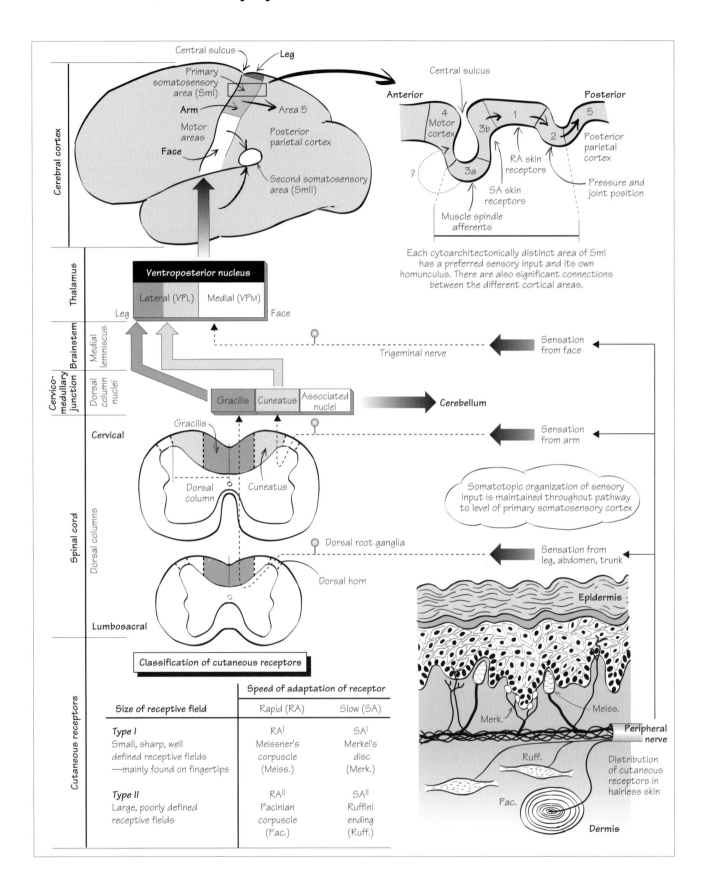

Each cytoarchitectonically distinct area of SmI has a preferred sensory input and its own homunculus. There are also significant connections between the different cortical areas.

Somatotopic organization of sensory input is maintained throughout pathway to level of primary somatosensory cortex

Classification of cutaneous receptors

Size of receptive field	Speed of adaptation of receptor	
	Rapid (RA)	Slow (SA)
Type I Small, sharp, well defined receptive fields —mainly found on fingertips	RA^I Meissner's corpuscle (Meiss.)	SA^I Merkel's disc (Merk.)
Type II Large, poorly defined receptive fields	RA^{II} Pacinian corpuscle (Pac.)	SA^{II} Ruffini ending (Ruff.)

Distribution of cutaneous receptors in hairless skin

The somatosensory system is the part of the nervous system that is involved in the processes of touch, pressure, proprioception (or joint position sense; see also Chapter 33), pain and temperature perception (see Chapters 21 and 22).

Sensory receptors

The **receptors for touch** are specialized nerve endings located in the skin with their cell bodies in the dorsal root ganglia. They are found at particularly high density in the fingertips, while those for proprioception are found not only in the skin but also in the muscle and joints (see Chapter 33).

Skin receptors can best be characterized by their structure, location, receptive fields and speed of adaptation. Type I receptors (**Meissner's corpuscles** and **Merkel's discs**) are packed in high density at the fingertips and provide accurate information about the exact location of a felt stimulus. In contrast, the rapidly adapting (RA) **Pacinian corpuscles** convey vibration perception, while the more slowly adapting (SA) **Ruffini endings** sense the magnitude, direction and rate of change of tension in the skin and deeper tissues.

Dorsal column–medial lemniscal pathway

These receptors are specialized nerve endings and the fast conducting, large diameter axons forming this are found in peripheral nerves and project into the **dorsal horn** of the spinal cord. The **trigeminal sensory system** for the face has a similar organization. Each class of receptor has a specific pattern of passage through the dorsal horn, but all ultimately end up in the **dorsal column** (with the exception of the trigeminal system), where they are organized according to receptor type and body location (somatotopy; see Chapter 12). They then project ipsilaterally up to the dorsal column nuclei (consisting of the gracile and cuneate nuclei), where they make their first synapse, although it should be realized that many dorsal column axons synapse at other spinal sites.

The **dorsal column nuclei (DCN)** are a complex series of structures that lie at the cervicomedullary junction and send axons which immediately decussate to form **medial lemniscus** which projects to the thalamus. The DCN also project to other brainstem structures, as well as receiving an input from the primary somatosensory cortex (SmI).

The medial lemniscus projects to the **ventroposterior (VP) nucleus of the thalamus**, picking up the trigeminal system as it ascends. This latter projection synapses in the medial part of the VP nucleus (VPM) with the remainder of the tract terminating in the lateral nucleus (VPL). This medial lemniscal termination is in the form of an anteroposterior thalamic rod, where all the cells have a similar modality and peripheral location (e.g. index finger, RA type I receptors). The thalamic rod then projects to layer IV of the SmI and forms the basis of the cortical column (see also Chapter 15).

The **SmI** consists of four different areas (Brodmann's areas 3a, 3b, 1 and 2), each of which has a separate representation of the contralateral body surface, with the tongue being represented laterally and the feet medially. The cortical representation is proportional to the receptor density in the skin so, for example, the hand has a much greater representation than the trunk (the **sensory homunculus**).

Primary and secondary sensory cortices

Each cortical area within SmI has slightly different response properties with respect to the neurones found in these areas. As one moves posteriorly towards the posterior parietal cortex the response properties of the neurones become more complex, implying a higher level of cortical analysis. SmI projects not only back to the dorsal column nuclei but to the **posterior parietal cortex** and **second somatosensory area (SmII)**. This latter area is found in the lateral wall of the Sylvian sulcus and is important in tactile object recognition, while the posterior parietal cortex input from SmI is important in the attribution of significance to a sensory stimulus (see Chapter 30).

The primary somatosensory pathway has developed during evolution with the corticospinal tract (CoST), which has a selective role in the control of fine finger movements (see Chapters 34–36). These two systems act together in the process of 'active touch' by which we explore our environment. Both systems display a degree of plasticity even in adult life (see Chapters 35 and 47). This is in part made possible by somatotopic organization of the sensory pathway: adjacent areas of skin are represented in neighbouring parts of the sensory system, at least as far as SmI.

Clinical disorders of the somatosensory system

Damage to the receptors and their afferent fibres can occur in a large number of *peripheral neuropathies*. Patients typically complain of both paraesthesiae and numbness, often in association with alterations in proprioception especially if the dorsal root ganglion is involved (see Chapters 31 and 33).

Lesions to the dorsal columns in the spinal cord are described in Chapter 31. Damage to the somatosensory pathway above the level of the DCN produces a contralateral sensory loss that will involve the face if the lesion lies at or above the level of the upper brainstem.

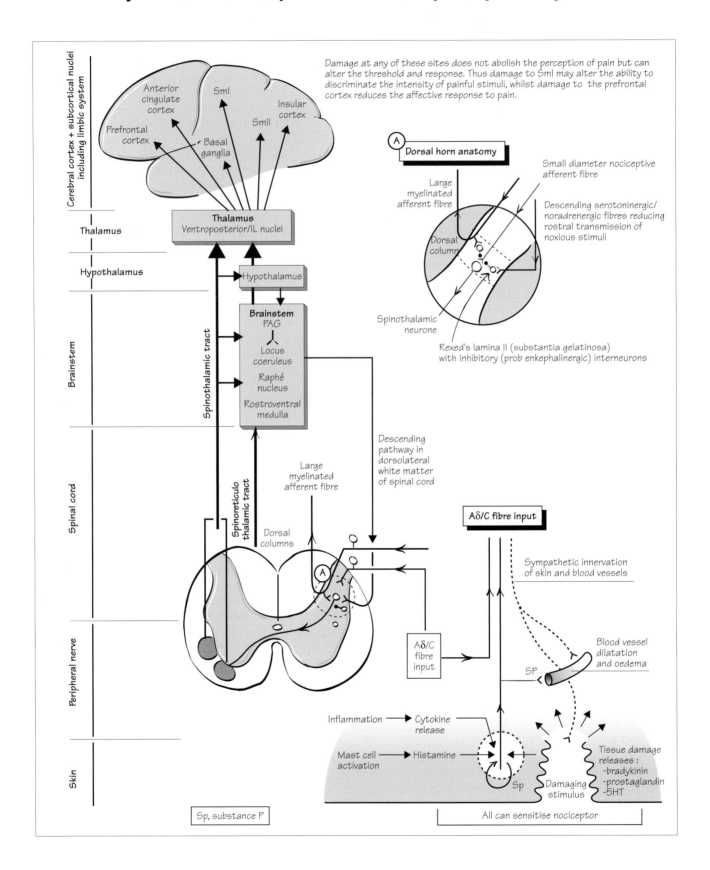

Damage at any of these sites does not abolish the perception of pain but can alter the threshold and response. Thus damage to SmI may alter the ability to discriminate the intensity of painful stimuli, whilst damage to the prefrontal cortex reduces the affective response to pain.

Cerebral cortex + subcortical nuclei including limbic system

Anterior cingulate cortex
SmI
Insular cortex
Prefrontal cortex
Basal ganglia
SmII

Thalamus
Thalamus
Ventroposterior/IL nuclei

Hypothalamus
Hypothalamus

Brainstem
Brainstem
PAG
Locus coeruleus
Raphé nucleus
Rostroventral medulla

Spinothalamic tract

Spinal cord
Spinoreticulo thalamic tract
Dorsal columns

Descending pathway in dorsolateral white matter of spinal cord

Large myelinated afferent fibre

Peripheral nerve

Skin

Aδ/C fibre input

A — Dorsal horn anatomy

Small diameter nociceptive afferent fibre

Large myelinated afferent fibre

Descending serotoninergic/ noradrenergic fibres reducing rostral transmission of noxious stimuli

Dorsal column

Spinothalamic neurone

Rexed's lamina II (substantia gelatinosa) with inhibitory (prob enkephalinergic) interneurons

Aδ/C fibre input

Sympathetic innervation of skin and blood vessels

Blood vessel dilatation and oedema

SP

Inflammation → Cytokine release

Mast cell activation → Histamine

Sp

Damaging stimulus

Tissue damage releases :
-bradykinin
-prostaglandin
-5HT

All can sensitise nociceptor

Sp, substance P

Pain is defined as an unpleasant sensory or emotional experience associated with actual or potential tissue damage or described in terms of such damage. Much of what is known about pain mechanisms has derived from animal-based research where the affective component is unclear and for this reason neuroscientists prefer to use the term **nociception** which defines the processing of information about damaging stimuli by the nervous system up to the point where perception occurs, probably at the level of the cerebral cortex. This is an important distinction because tissue damage is not inevitably linked to pain and in humans this can sometimes be seen with damaging injuries acquired in stressful situations such as in war.

Nociceptors

Nociceptors are found in the skin, visceral organs, skeletal and cardiac muscle and in association with blood vessels. They conduct information about noxious events to the dorsal horn of the spinal cord where the primary afferents synapse predominantly on interneurones as opposed to projection neurones.

There are basically two types of nociceptor distinguished by the diameter of the afferent fibre and the stimulus required to activate it. The **high-threshold mechanoreceptor (HTM)** is activated by intense mechanical stimulation and innervated by **thinly myelinated Aδ fibres** conducting at 5–30 m/s. **Polymodal nociceptors (PMN)** respond to intense mechanical stimulation, temperatures in excess of about 42°C and irritant chemicals. These receptors are innervated by **unmyelinated C fibres** conducting at 0.5–2 m/s. Sharply localized pain is thought to be conducted in the faster conducting fibres whereas poorly localized pain may be conducted in the C fibres.

Although nociceptors are histologically simple free nerve endings, the process of **transduction** at the receptor ending is complex and is associated with some of the chemical mediators of inflammation and tissue damage. Thus, adenosine triphosphate (ATP), bradykinin, histamine and prostaglandins all either activate or sensitize the receptor ending and indeed some of the transmitters in the nociceptive pathway are themselves released peripherally (e.g. substance P) to produce further sensitization of the receptor ending. This receptor sensitization helps to explain the perception of heightened pain (**primary hyperalgesia**) in areas of tissue damage, but it does not fully explain the perception of non-painful stimuli as painful (**allodynia or secondary hyperalgesia**) in cases of peripheral or central nerve damage. In this respect recent evidence suggests that both allodynia and some chronic pain syndromes (e.g. phantom limb pain) are caused by long-term changes in the processing of noxious information in the dorsal horn of the spinal cord. Visceral nociceptors project into the spinal cord via the small-diameter myelinated and unmyelinated fibres of the autonomic nervous system, and synapse at the spinal level of their embryological origin. The development of pain in an internal organ can therefore produce the perception of a painful stimulus in the skin rather than the organ itself, at least in the early stages of inflammation—a phenomenon known as **referred pain**. For example, inflammation of the appendix initially leads to pain being perceived at the umbilicus.

Nociceptive pathways

The majority of nociceptors and thermoreceptors project into the spinal cord via the dorsal root, although some pass through the ventral horn. On reaching the spinal cord these sensory nerves synapse in a complex fashion in the dorsal horn.

At this site, changes in synaptic transmission can occur. Indeed, the arrival of axonally conducted substance P in the superficial layers of the dorsal horn leads to both an increase in receptive field sizes and the sensitivity of some dorsal horn neurones. These functional changes are also mediated in part by the synaptic release of glutamate acting on post-synaptic N-methyl-D-aspartate (NMDA) receptors. These long-term changes are examples of neuronal plasticity (see Chapter 47) and in the context of the dorsal horn contribute to some chronic pain states.

The postsynaptic cell conveying nociceptive information projects up the spinal cord as the **spinothalamic**, **spinoreticulothalamic** and **spinomesencephalic** tracts (latter not shown on figure), with the axons crossing at the spinal level by passing around the central canal of the cord. This crossing of fibres often occurs a few levels above where the nociceptive fibres enter the cord, and thus damage in the region of the central canal as occurs in *syringomyelia* leads to a loss of pain and temperature sensibility in a dermatomal distribution often several levels below the site of the lesion (see Chapter 31).

The postsynaptic cell and presynaptic nociceptive nerve terminal receive synapses from other peripherally projecting somatosensory systems, descending projections from the brainstem and interneurones intrinsic to the dorsal horn. Many of these interneurones contain **endogenous opioid substances** known as enkephalins and endorphins which activate opioid receptors of which there are three main subtypes (μ, κ, δ). There is therefore enormous potential for modifying the transfer of nociceptive information at the level of the dorsal horn (see Chapter 22).

The **ascending nociceptive pathways** synapse in a number of different central nervous system (CNS) sites. Information concerning noxious events ascends in either the spinothalamic tract (providing accurate localization) or the spinoreticulothalamic system (transmitting information concerning the affective components of pain). However, some of the nuclei in the brainstem to which these pathways project (e.g. the raphe nucleus and locus ceruleus) in turn send axons back down the spinal cord to the dorsal horn, and can be exploited in the control of chronic pain syndromes (see Chapter 22).

The thalamic termination of the spinothalamic pathway is in the ventoposterior and intralaminar nuclei (IL) (including the posterior group), which in turn project to multiple cortical areas but especially the primary somatosensory cortex (SmI) and second somatosensory area (SmII) and the anterior cingulate cortex. However, other areas receive an input from these nuclei including the prefrontal cortex, basal ganglia and insular cortex. Lesions to any of these sites alter the perception of pain but do not produce a true and complete loss of pain or analgesia, and indeed may even produce a chronic pain syndrome. Such syndromes are not uncommonly seen with small thalamic cerebrovascular accidents.

The thermoreceptors, and to a lesser extent the nociceptors, also project to the hypothalamus which has an important role in thermoregulation, and the autonomic response to a painful stimulus (see Chapters 42 and 43).

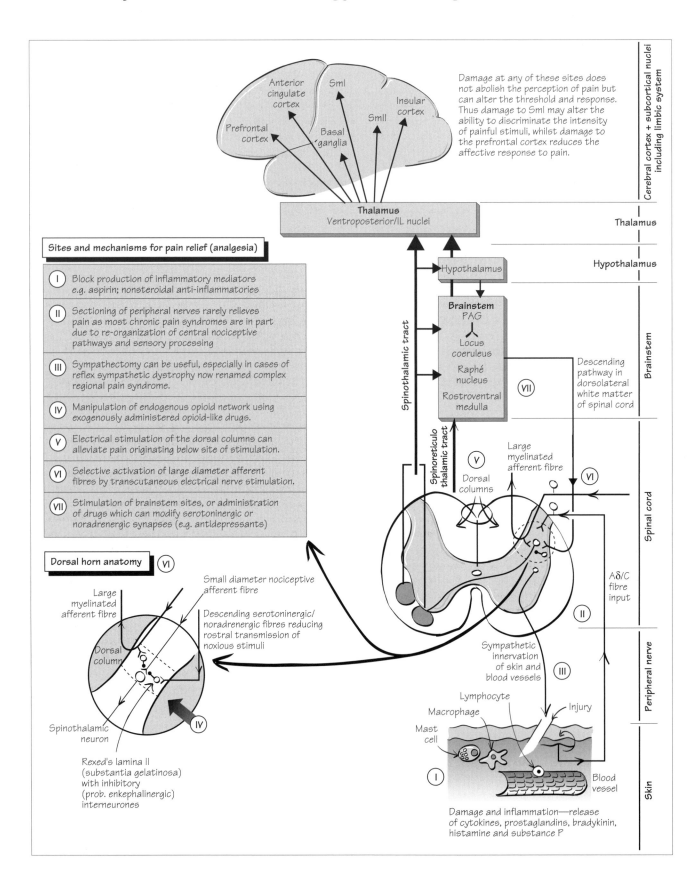

Cerebral cortex + subcortical nuclei including limbic system

Damage at any of these sites does not abolish the perception of pain but can alter the threshold and response. Thus damage to Sml may alter the ability to discriminate the intensity of painful stimuli, whilst damage to the prefrontal cortex reduces the affective response to pain.

Anterior cingulate cortex

Sml

Insular cortex

Prefrontal cortex

Basal ganglia

Smll

Thalamus
Ventroposterior/IL nuclei

Thalamus

Hypothalamus

Hypothalamus

Sites and mechanisms for pain relief (analgesia)

Ⓘ Block production of inflammatory mediators e.g. aspirin; nonsteroidal anti-inflammatories

Ⓘⓘ Sectioning of peripheral nerves rarely relieves pain as most chronic pain syndromes are in part due to re-organization of central nociceptive pathways and sensory processing

Ⓘⓘⓘ Sympathectomy can be useful, especially in cases of reflex sympathetic dystrophy now renamed complex regional pain syndrome.

Ⓘⓥ Manipulation of endogenous opioid network using exogenously administered opioid-like drugs.

Ⓥ Electrical stimulation of the dorsal columns can alleviate pain originating below site of stimulation.

Ⓥⓘ Selective activation of large diameter afferent fibres by transcutaneous electrical nerve stimulation.

Ⓥⓘⓘ Stimulation of brainstem sites, or administration of drugs which can modify serotoninergic or noradrenergic synapses (e.g. antidepressants)

Brainstem
PAG

Locus coeruleus

Raphé nucleus

Rostroventral medulla

Ⓥⓘⓘ

Descending pathway in dorsolateral white matter of spinal cord

Brainstem

Spinothalamic tract

Spinoreticulo thalamic tract

Ⓥ Dorsal columns

Large myelinated afferent fibre

Ⓥⓘ

Dorsal horn anatomy Ⓥⓘ

Aδ/C fibre input

Ⓘⓘ

Spinal cord

Large myelinated afferent fibre

Small diameter nociceptive afferent fibre

Descending serotoninergic/ noradrenergic fibres reducing rostral transmission of noxious stimuli

Dorsal column

Spinothalamic neuron

Ⓘⓥ

Rexed's lamina II (substantia gelatinosa) with inhibitory (prob. enkephalinergic) interneurones

Sympathetic innervation of skin and blood vessels

Ⓘⓘⓘ

Lymphocyte

Macrophage

Mast cell

Injury

Ⓘ

Blood vessel

Peripheral nerve

Skin

Damage and inflammation—release of cytokines, prostaglandins, bradykinin, histamine and substance P

The development of pain is a common experience and the treatment for it is important not only where it is caused by injury or inflammation but also in cases where the nerves themselves are damaged (e.g. neuropathies). In these latter cases the pain can arise from a site of previous injury or may develop for more obscure reasons (e.g. *reflex sympathetic dystrophy*, now renamed *complex regional pain syndrome*). In all cases the development of pain is both disabling and depressing and a multidisciplinary approach is often needed involving psychologists as well as pain specialists and pharmacological measures.

Management of pain

Pain relief or analgesia can be approached using a number of different strategies. Many analgesic therapies work by reducing the peripheral inflammatory response which is also responsible for receptor sensitization (**Site I** on figure). The interruption of peripheral nerve conduction by the injection of local anaesthetics can be helpful in some pain states, but lesioning of the peripheral nerve is usually without effect in ameliorating neuropathic pain (**Site II**). However, in some cases nerve injury results in the formation of a neuroma which consists of scar tissue and aborted axonal regeneration (see Chapter 46). This in turn leads to the generation of abnormal signals within the injured nerve that are perceived as painful. In such circumstances local excision of the neuroma may benefit the patient.

The organization of the nociceptive input to the dorsal horn has been explored clinically in pain management. For example, stimulation of non-nociceptive receptors can inhibit the transmission of nociceptive information in the dorsal horn, which means that painful stimuli can be 'gated' out by counter irritation using non-painful stimuli. This is the basis of the **gate theory** of Wall and Melzack and is exploited clinically by the use of transcutaneous nerve stimulation (TENS) in areas of pain (**Site VI**), as well as the stimulation of the dorsal columns themselves in some cases of chronic pain (**Site V**). Similarly, the supraspinal input can also gate out noxious stimuli when activated (**Site VII**), as occurs in stressful situations when attending to a painful stimulus would not necessarily be useful (e.g. war injuries). These supraspinal nuclei can also be manipulated pharmacologically, with the administration of drugs that are normally used in the treatment of depression (see Chapter 50). These antidepressant drugs with a presumed action at the noradrenergic and serotoninergic synapse have been used to treat pain states, irrespective of any antidepressant action they might have (**Site VII**). The most commonly used agents are amine uptake inhibitors, such as imipramine and amitriptyline (tricyclic antidepressants). These agents appear to alter the pain threshold but are not without side-effects because they have blocking actions on muscarinic receptors (dry mouth, constipation, blurred vision), α-adrenoceptors (postural hypotension) and histamine H_1-receptors (sedation).

Furthermore, the recognition that one of the major transmitters in the nociceptive pathway is substance P (SP) has led to the development of other analgesic medications. For example, capsaicin (the active ingredient of red chilli), which initially releases SP from nociceptors and subsequently inactivates the SP-containing C fibres, can be used topically in some pain syndromes such as *postherpetic neuralgia*. However, perhaps the most common exploitation of this system medically is the manipulation of the enkephalinergic interneurone and opioid receptors by the exogenous administration of morphine and its analogues to control pain (**Site IV**).

Opioid analgesics are drugs that mimic endogenous opioid peptides by causing a prolonged activation of opioid receptors (usually μ-receptors). This reduces pain transmission at synapses in the dorsal horn of the spinal cord by an inhibitory action on the relay neurones. Opioids also stimulate noradrenergic, serotoninergic and enkephalinergic neurones in the brainstem that descend in the spinal cord and further inhibit the relay neurones of the spinothalamic tract. Opioid analgesics are widely used to relieve dull, poorly localized (visceral) pain. Repeated doses may cause dependence. In drug addicts, the dose necessary to cause euphoria may rapidly increase (tolerance) but in patients the necessity for higher dosage usually reflects progressively increasing pain.

Morphine is the most widely used analgesic in severe pain but, like all strong opioids, may cause nausea and vomiting. Other effects of morphine-type drugs include euphoria, respiratory depression, constipation and pinpoint pupils caused by stimulation of the third nerve nucleus. Other opioids used in severe pain include diamorphine (heroin), pethidine and methadone. Codeine and dextropropoxyphene are weaker drugs used in mild to moderate pain. **Naloxone** is an antagonist at opioid receptors and is used to reverse the effects of opioid overdose.

Furthermore, although pain typically arises from tissue damage, it can also occur with damage to the peripheral (PNS) and central (CNS) nervous systems. One such example is trigeminal neuralgia, which is characterized by paroxysms of facial pain. In this condition the patient experiences paroxysms of pain in one of the three divisions of the trigeminal nerve and although in the majority of cases the cause of the condition is not found, it can be seen in some people with *multiple sclerosis*. It can be treated surgically by lesioning of the appropriate nerve root, although most cases respond to the antiepileptic agent carbamazepine or gabapentin (see Chapter 53). Another example of a pain syndrome arising with damage to neural tissue is seen following trauma to a peripheral nerve trunk, where a change in autonomic innervation to the traumatized limb results in the development of severe pain *(reflex sympathetic dystrophies)*. The reason for the development of such states is not known, although the nociceptive nerve endings do appear to start expressing receptors for noradrenaline. Thus, local sympathectomies can be helpful in alleviating this pain, although this is not always the case (**Site III**).

23 The visual system I: The eye and retina

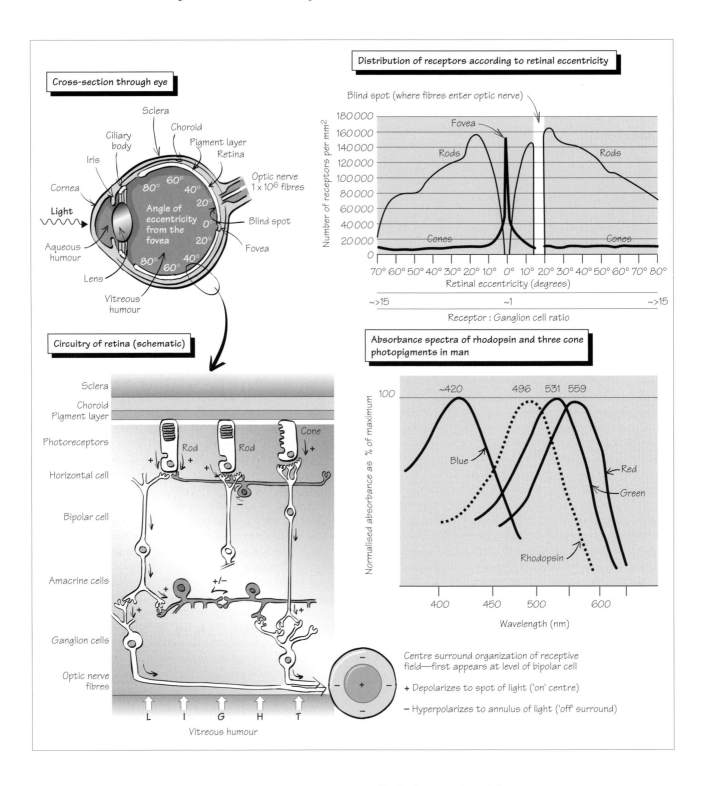

The visual system is responsible for converting all incident light energy into a visual image of the world. This information is coded for in the retina which lies at the back of the eye, and then transmits that information to the visual cortical areas, the hypothalamus and upper brainstem (see Chapters 24 and 25). The process of visual transduction is detailed in Chapter 19.

Optical properties of the eye

On reaching the eye, light has to be precisely focused on to the retina, and this process of **refraction** is dependent on the curvature of the cornea and the axial length of the eye. Failure to do this accurately leads to either an inability to see clearly when reading (*long-sight or hypermetropia*), or to see distant objects clearly (*short-sight or myopia*), or both. In the latter case there is often an additional problem of *astigmatism*, in which the refraction of the eye varies in different meridians.

In addition to the need to be refracted precisely on to the retina, light must also be transmitted without any loss of quality and this relies on the cornea, anterior and posterior chambers and lens all being clear. Injuries or disease of any of these components can lead to a reduced **visual acuity** (the ability to discriminate detail). The most common conditions affecting these parts of the eye are infections and damage to the cornea *(keratitis)* or opacification of the lens *(cataracts)*.

Retinal anatomy and function

The light on striking the **retina** is transduced into electrical signals by the **photoreceptors** that lie on the innermost layer of the retina, furthest from the vitreous humour. There are two main types of photoreceptors: **rods and cones**. The rods are found in all areas of the retina, except the fovea, and are sensitive to low levels of light and are thus responsible for our vision at night **(scotopic vision)**. Many rods relay their information to a single ganglion cell, and so this system is sensitive to absolute levels of illumination while not being capable of discriminating fine visual detail and colour. Thus, at night we can detect objects but not in any detail or colour.

The cones are found at highest density in the **fovea** and contain one of three different **photopigments**. They are responsible for our daytime or **photopic vision**. This, coupled to the high density of these receptors at the **fovea**, where they have an almost one-to-one relationship with ganglion cells, means that they are the receptors responsible for visual acuity and colour vision. Alterations in the photopigments contained within these receptors leads to *colour blindness*. Diseases of the receptors leading to their death, such as *retinitis pigmentosa*, lead to a progressive loss of vision that typically affects the peripheral retina and rods in the early stages, resulting in night blindness and constricted visual fields.

The photoreceptors make synapses with both horizontal and bipolar cells. The **horizontal cells** have two major roles: (i) they create the centre surround organization of the receptive field of the bipolar cell; and (ii) they are responsible for shifting the spectral sensitivity of the bipolar cell to match the level of background illumination (part of the light adaptation response; see Chapter 19). The **centre surround receptive field** means that a bipolar cell will respond to a small spot of light in the middle of its receptive field in one way (depolarization or hyperpolarization), while an annulus or ring of light around that central spot of light will produce an opposite response. The horizontal cells, by receiving inputs from many receptors and synapsing on to the photoreceptor bipolar cell, can provide the necessary information for this receptive field to be generated. The mechanism by which they fulfil their other role in light adaptation is not fully understood.

The **bipolar cells** relay information from the photoreceptors to the ganglion cells and receive synapses from photoreceptors, horizontal and amacrine cells. They can be classified according to the receptor they receive from (cone only, rod only, or both) or their response to light. Bipolar cells that are hyperpolarized by a small spot of light in the centre of their receptive fields are termed **off-centre (on-surround)** while the converse is true for those bipolar cells that are depolarized by a small spot of light in the centre of their receptive field.

The **ganglion cells** are found closest to the vitreous humour, receive from both bipolar and amacrine cells and send their axons to the brain via the optic nerve. These nerve fibres course over the inner surface of the retina before leaving at a site which forms the **optic disc** and which is responsible for the **blind spot** as no receptors are located at this site. This blind spot is not usually apparent in normal vision. The ganglion cells can be classified in a number of different ways: according to their morphology; their response to light as for bipolar cells ('on' or 'off' centre); or a combination of these properties (the **XYW system**). The X ganglion cells, which make up 80% of the retinal ganglion cell population, are involved in the analysis of detail and colour while the Y ganglion cells are more involved in motion detection. The W ganglion cells, which make up the remaining 10% of the population, project to the brainstem but as yet have no clearly defined function. The X and Y ganglion cell system defined initially in cats is equivalent to the P and M channel in primates, which is broadly responsible for 'form' and 'movement' coding, respectively.

The **amacrine cells** of the retina, which make up the final class of retinal cells, receive and relay signals from and to bipolar cells, other amacrine cells and ganglion cells. There are many different types of amacrine cells, some of which are exclusively related to rods and others to cones, and they contain a number of different transmitters. They tend to have complex responses to light stimuli and are important in generating many of the response properties of ganglion cells, including the detection and coding of moving objects and the onset and offset of illumination.

24 The visual system II: The visual pathways and subcortical visual areas

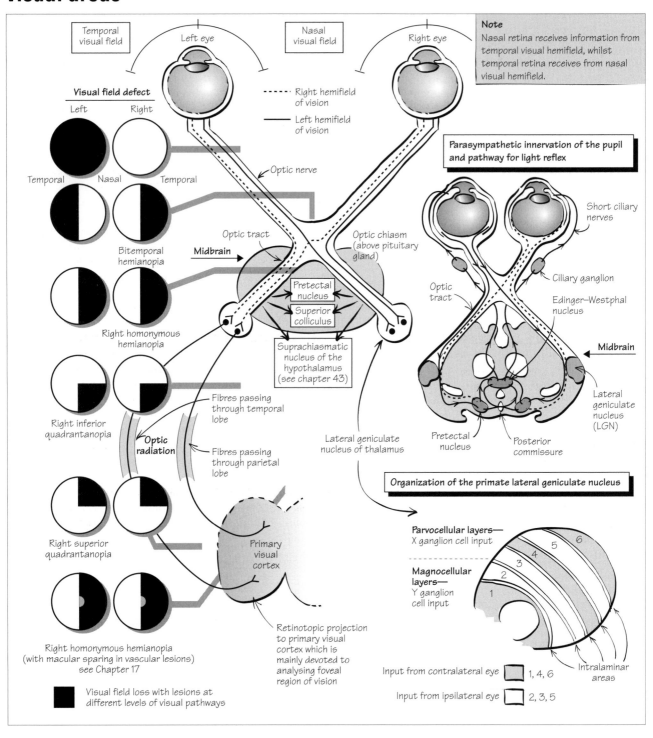

The **retina** conveys its information from the ganglion cells to a number of different sites, including several cortical areas via the thalamus, the hypothalamus and midbrain. The major cortical projection is via the lateral geniculate nucleus (LGN) of the thalamus to the primary visual cortex (V1 or Brodmann's area 17). Other cortical areas (known collec-

tively as the extrastriate areas) receive information from the LGN as well as the pulvinar region of the thalamus (see Chapter 25).

The projection from the retina to V1 maintains its retinotopic organization, such that a lesion along the course of the pathway produces a predictable visual field defect. Lesions in front of the optic chiasm typically produce uniocular field defects while lesions of the chiasm (e.g. from pituitary tumours) cause a bitemporal hemianopia. Lesions behind the chiasm typically produce similar field defects in both eyes, e.g. a homonymous hemianopia or quandrantanopia.

Lateral geniculate nucleus

The **LGN** consists of six layers in primates, with each layer receiving an input from either the ipsilateral or contralateral eye. The inner two with their large neurones form the magnocellular laminae while the remaining four layers constitute the parvocellular laminae. The morphological distinction between the neurones in these two laminae is also found electrophysiologically.

The parvocellular neurones display chromatic or colour sensitivity and sensitivity to high spatial frequency (detail) with sustained responses to visual stimuli. In contrast, the magnocellular neurones show no colour selectivity, respond best to low spatial frequencies and often have a transient response on being stimulated. Thus, the magnocellular layer neurones have similar properties to the Y ganglion cells and the parvocellular neurones to the X ganglion cells, a similarity that is reflected in the retinogeniculate projection of these two classes of ganglion cells. The X ganglion cells and the parvocellular laminae neurones are responsible for the detection of colour and form (or *Pattern*) and constitute the **P channel**, while the **M channel** of the Y ganglion cells and the magnocellular laminae of the LGN are responsible primarily for motion detection (or *Movement*).

The LGN mainly projects to the **V1** where the afferent fibres synapse in layer IV, and to a lesser extent layer VI, with the M and P channels having different synaptic targets within these laminae. In addition, there is a projection from cells that lie between the laminae of the LGN (intralaminar part of the LGN) direct to layers II and III of V1 (see Chapter 25).

Superior colliculus

The superior colliculus in the midbrain is a multilayered structure, wherein the superficial layers are involved in mapping the visual field and the deep layers with complex sensory integration involving visual, auditory and somatosensory stimuli. The intermediate layers are involved in saccadic eye movements and receive connections from the occipitoparietal cortex, the frontal eye fields and the substantia nigra (see Chapter 40). The saccadic eye movements are tightly mapped in the superior colliculus, so that stimulation at a given point within it will cause a saccadic eye movement to bring the point of fixation to that point in the visual field which is represented in the more superficial layers of this structure. This ability to line up different sensorimotor representations in the superior colliculus in register even extends down into the deeper layers. In other words, a vertical descent through this structure encounters, in order: (i) neurones that respond to visual stimuli in a given part of the visual field; (ii) neurones that cause saccadic eye movements which bring the fovea to bear on to that same part of the visual scene; (iii) auditory and somatosensory neurones that are maximally activated by sounds that originate from that part of the environment and by areas of skin that would most likely be activated by a physical contact with an object located in that part of the extrapersonal space. This latter feature accounts for the fact that in the superior colliculus the somatosensory representation is primarily skewed towards the nose and face. Thus, the superior colliculus not only codes for saccades, but tends to code specifically for those saccades that are triggered by stimuli of behavioural significance as well as having a more widespread function in orienting responses. This role for the superior colliculus is reflected in its efferent connections to a number of brainstem structures as well as the spinal cord (tectospinal tract). Clinically, damage is rarely confined to this structure but when it is there is a profound loss of saccadic eye movements with neglect.

Pretectal structures and the pupillary response to light

There is a projection from the optic tract to the pretectal nuclei of the midbrain which in turn projects bilaterally to the Edinger–Westphal nucleus which provides the parasympathetic input to the pupil allowing it to constrict. Light shone in one eye will cause constriction of both pupils (direct and consensual response). Damage to one of the optic nerves will cause a reduced direct and consensual response but that same eye will constrict normally to light shone in the unaffected eye, producing a *relative afferent pupillary defect*.

Suprachiasmatic nucleus of the hypothalamus

This nucleus receives a direct retinal input and is important in the generation and control of circadian rhythms (see Chapter 43).

25 The visual system III: Visual cortical areas

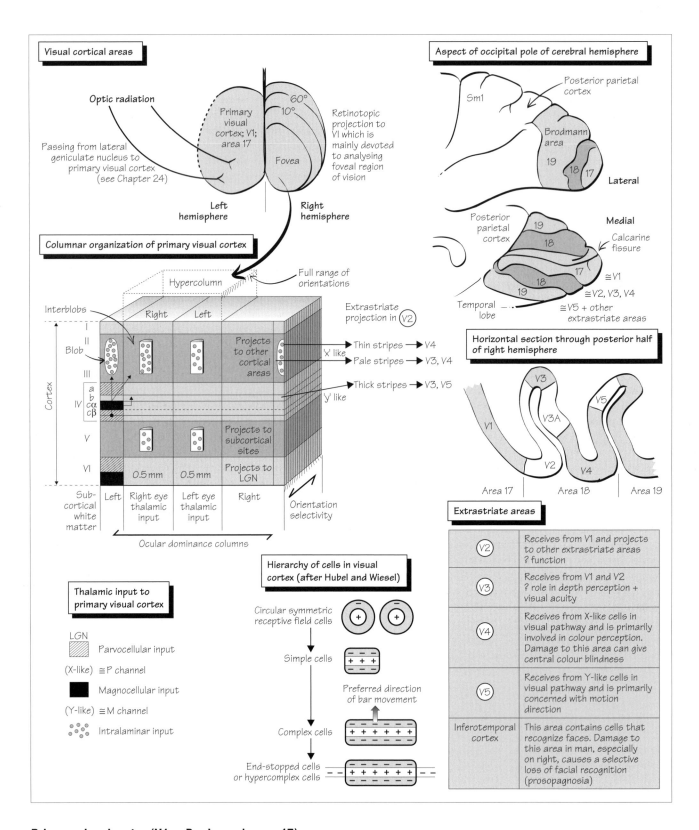

Primary visual cortex (V1 or Brodmann's area 17)

The primary visual cortex (V1) lies along the calcarine fissure of the occipital lobe and receives its major input from the lateral geniculate nucleus (LGN). These connections are organized **retinotopically** so that adjacent areas of the retina project up the visual pathway via neighbouring axons. This retinal projection is, however, not a simple map, as the critical factor is the relationship of the photoreceptors to the projecting ganglion cell of the retina. This means that the centre of vision (especially the fovea) dominates the retinal projection to V1 because of the near one-to-one relationship of photoreceptor to ganglion cell at the fovea in contrast to the peripheral retina (see Chapter 23).

The LGN projection to V1 is mainly to layer IV and is different for the M and P channels, while the projection from the intralaminar part of the LGN is to layers II and III of V1 (see below). The LGN input to layer IV of V1 is so great that this cortical layer is futher subdivided into IVa, IVb, IVcα and IVcβ, with each subdivision having slightly different connections. However, in general the cortical neurones in layer IVc of V1 have **centre surround or circular symmetric receptive field organization** (see Chapter 23). These layer IVc neurones then project on to other adjacent neurones within the cortex, in such a way that several neurones of this type converge on to a single neurone whose receptive field is now more complex in terms of the stimulus that best activates it. These cells respond most effectively to a line or bar of illumination of a given orientation and are termed **simple cells**. These cells in turn project in a convergent fashion on to other neurones (**complex cells**), which are predominantly found in layers II and III, and which are maximally activated by stimuli of a given orientation moving in a particular direction, that direction often being orthogonal to the line orientation.

The complex cells project to the **hypercomplex or end-stopped cells** which respond to a line of a given orientation and length. This series of cells originally described by Hubel and Wiesel are thus organized in a hierarchical fashion, with each cell deriving its receptive field from the cells immediately beneath it in the hierarchy.

Hubel and Wiesel further discovered that these neurones were organized into columns of cells with similar properties; the two properties that they originally studied being the eye that provides the dominant input to that neurone (giving **ocular dominance columns**) and the orientation of the line needed to activate neurones maximally (giving **orientation selective columns**). They represented these two sets of columns as running orthogonal to each other, and the area of cortex containing an ocular dominance column from each eye with a complete set of orientation selective columns being termed the **hypercolumn**. This hypercolumn, which is 1 mm^2 in size, is capable of analysing a given section of the visual field that is defined by the corresponding retinal inputs from both eyes. In the case of the fovea, where there is near unity of photoreceptors to ganglion cells, this visual field is very small, while the converse is true for more peripheral retinal inputs. Therefore a shift of 1 mm in the cortex from one hypercolumn to another leads to a shift in the location of the visual field being analysed, with most of these being concerned with foveal vision (see below).

However, there are two main major complicating factors with this model. One is the accommodation of the M and P channels and the second relates to the discovery of cytochrome oxidase (a marker of metabolic activity) -rich areas in layers II, III and IVb (and, to a lesser extent, layers V and VI) which show no orientation selectivity but colour and high spatial frequency sensitivity. These cytochrome oxidase-rich areas in layers II and III are grouped together to form **'blobs'**, at least one of which is associated with each ocular dominance column, with the areas between them being termed **interblobs**. Both the blobs and interblobs, together with the cytochrome-rich layer IVb, have distinct projections to V2 and other extrastriate areas—projections that correlate well with the M and P channels. This arrangement of channels and connections suggests that visual information is not so much processed in a hierarchical fashion, but by a series of parallel pathways (see Chapter 15).

The major function of V1, apart from being the first site of binocular interactions, is to deconstruct the visual field into small line segments of various orientation as well as segregating and integrating components of the visual image which can then be relayed to more specialist visual areas. These areas perform more complex visual analysis but rely on their interaction with V1 for the conscious perception of the whole visual image. This occasionally presents itself clinically in patients with bilateral damage to V1, in which they deny being able to see any visual stimulus even though on formal testing they are capable of localizing visual targets accurately (a phenomenon known as *blindsight*).

Visual association or extrastriate areas

The **extrastriate areas** are those cortical areas outside V1 that are primarily involved in visual processing. The number of such areas varies from species to species, with the greatest number being found in humans. These areas are found within Brodmann's areas 18 and 19 and the inferotemporal cortex and are involved in more complex visual processing than V1, with one aspect of the visual scene tending to be dominant in terms of the analysis undertaken by that cortical area (e.g. colour or motion detection). In addition, there are a number of other parts of the CNS that are associated with the visual system including the **posterior parietal cortex** (see Chapter 30); **the frontal cortex and frontal eye fields** (see Chapters 30 and 40); and the subcortical structures of the **hypothalamus** (see Chapter 43) and **upper brainstem** (see Chapter 24).

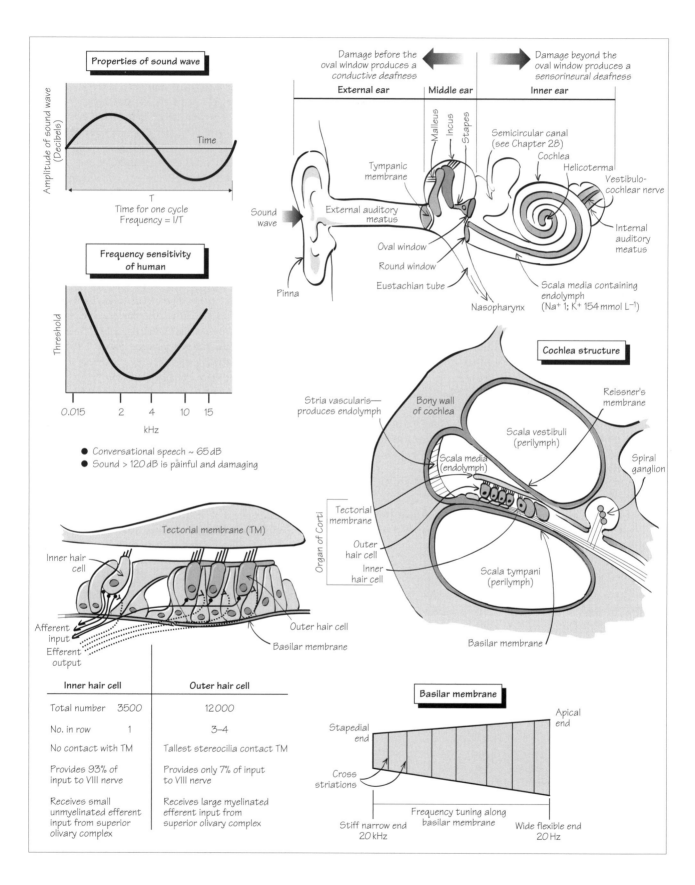

Properties of sound wave

Amplitude of sound wave (Decibels)

Time

Time for one cycle
Frequency = 1/T

Frequency sensitivity of human

Threshold

0.015 2 4 10 15

kHz

- Conversational speech ~ 65 dB
- Sound > 120 dB is painful and damaging

Damage before the oval window produces a conductive deafness

Damage beyond the oval window produces a sensorineural deafness

| External ear | Middle ear | Inner ear |

Malleus
Incus
Stapes

Tympanic membrane

Semicircular canal (see Chapter 28)

Cochlea

Helicoterma

Vestibulo-cochlear nerve

Sound wave

External auditory meatus

Oval window

Round window

Eustachian tube

Nasopharynx

Pinna

Internal auditory meatus

Scala media containing endolymph
(Na+ 1; K+ 154 mmol L⁻¹)

Cochlea structure

Stria vascularis— produces endolymph

Bony wall of cochlea

Reissner's membrane

Scala vestibuli (perilymph)

Scala media (endolymph)

Spiral ganglion

Tectorial membrane

Outer hair cell

Inner hair cell

Organ of Corti

Scala tympani (perilymph)

Basilar membrane

Tectorial membrane (TM)

Inner hair cell

Afferent input

Efferent output

Outer hair cell

Basilar membrane

	Inner hair cell	Outer hair cell
Total number	3500	12 000
No. in row	1	3–4
	No contact with TM	Tallest stereocilia contact TM
	Provides 93% of input to VIII nerve	Provides only 7% of input to VIII nerve
	Receives small unmyelinated efferent input from superior olivary complex	Receives large myelinated efferent input from superior olivary complex

Basilar membrane

Apical end

Stapedial end

Cross striations

Frequency tuning along basilar membrane

Stiff narrow end 20 kHz

Wide flexible end 20 Hz

The **auditory system** is responsible for sound perception. The receptive end-organ is the cochlea of the inner ear which converts sound waves into electrical signals by a process of mechanotransduction. The electrical signal generated in response to a sound is passed (together with information from the vestibular system; see Chapter 28) via the eighth cranial nerve (vestibulocochlear nerve) to the brainstem where it synapses in the cochlear nuclear complex (see Chapter 27).

Although the auditory system as a whole performs many functions, the primary site responsible for frequency discrimination is at the level of the cochlea.

Properties of sound waves

A **sound wave** is characterized by its **amplitude** or **loudness** (measured in decibels (dB)), **frequency** or **pitch** (measured in hertz (Hz)), **waveform**, **phase** and **quality** or **timbre**. The intensity of sound can vary enormously but in general we can discriminate changes in intensity of around 1–2 dB.

The arrival of a sound at the head creates phase and intensity differences between the two ears unless the sound originates from the midline. The degree of delay and intensity change between the two ears as a result of their physical separation is useful but probably not necessary for the localization of sounds (see Chapter 27).

External and middle ear

On reaching the ear the sound passes down the **external auditory meatus** to the **tympanic membrane or eardrum**, which vibrates at a frequency and strength determined by the impinging sound. This causes the **three ear ossicles** in the **middle ear** to move, displacing fluid within the **cochlea** as the stapedial foot process moves within the oval window of the cochlea. This process is essential in reducing the acoustic impedance of the system and in enhancing the response to sound, because a sound hitting a fluid directly is largely reflected.

There are two small muscles associated with the ear ossicles, which protect them from damage by loud noises as well as modifying the movement of the stapedial foot process in the oval window. Damage to the ear ossicles (e.g. *otosclerosis*), middle ear (e.g. infection or *otitis media*) or external auditory meatus (e.g. blockage by wax) all lead to a reduction in hearing or *deafness* that is **conductive** in nature.

Inner ear and cochlea

The displacement of the stapedial foot process in the **oval window** gen-erates waves in the perilymph-filled scala vestibuli and tympani of the cochlea. These two scalae are in communication at the apical end of the cochlea, the helicotrema, but are separated for the rest of their length by the scala media that contains the transduction apparatus in the organ of Corti.

The organ of Corti sits on the floor of the scala media on a structure known as the **basilar membrane (BM)**, the width of which increases with distance from the stapedial end. This increase in width coupled to a decrease in stiffness of the BM means that sounds of high frequency maximally displace the BM at the stapedial end of the cochlea while low-frequency sounds maximally activate the apical end of the BM. Thus, frequency tuning is, in part, a function of the BM although it is greatly enhanced and made more selective by the hair cells of the organ of Corti that lie on this membrane.

The **organ of Corti** is a complex structure that contains the cells of **auditory transduction**, the **hair cells** (see Chapter 19), which are of two types in this structure: a single row of inner hair cells (IHCs) that provide most of the signal in the eighth cranial nerve; and 3–4 rows of outer hair cells (OHCs) that have a role in modulating the response of IHCs to a given sound. These two types of hair cells are morphologically and electrophysiologically distinct. While the IHCs receive little input from the brainstem, the OHCs do so in the form of an input from the superior olivary complex which has the effect of modifying the shape and response properties of these cells. Some of the OHCs make direct contact with the overlying **tectorial membrane (TM)** in the organ of Corti which may be important in modifying the response of the IHCs to sound, as these cells do not contact the TM but do provide 93% of the afferent input of the cochlear nerve. One afferent fibre receives from many OHCs, but a single IHC is associated with many afferent fibres. In addition to these differences between OHCs and IHCs, there are subtle alterations in the hair cells themselves with distance along the scala media. These alterations in shape alter their tuning characteristics which adds a degree of refinement to frequency tuning, beyond that imparted by the resonance properties of the BM.

Damage to the cochlea, hair cells or cochlear part of the vestibulocochlear nerve leads to *deafness* that is described as being **sensorineural** in nature. Trauma, ischaemia and tumours of the eighth cranial nerve can all cause this. Certain hereditary causes of deafness have been associated recently with defects in the proteins found in the stereocilia of hair cells.

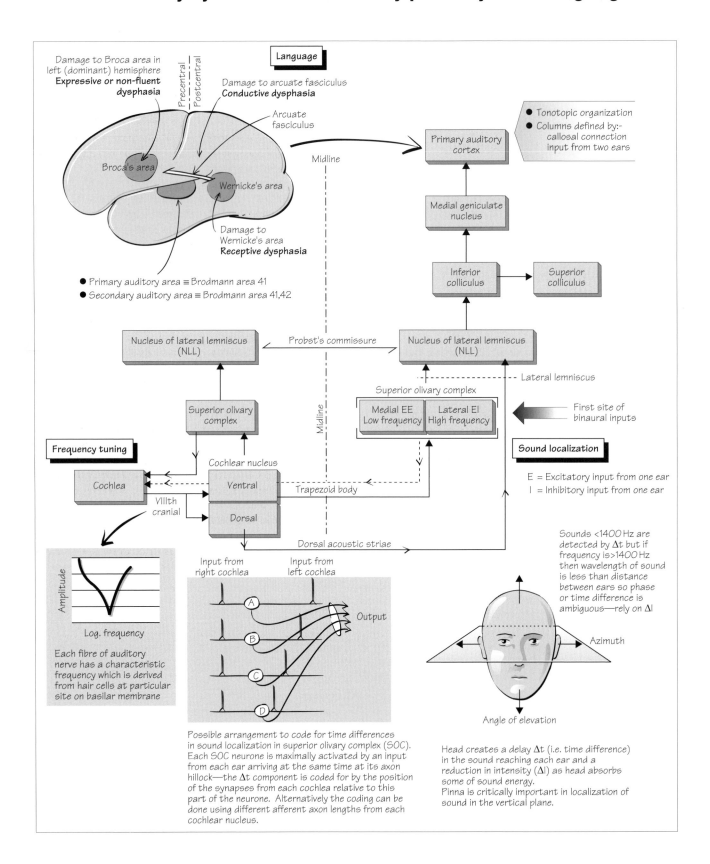

Damage to Broca area in left (dominant) hemisphere **Expressive or non-fluent dysphasia**

Damage to arcuate fasciculus **Conductive dysphasia**

Arcuate fasciculus

Precentral
Postcentral

Language

Broca's area

Wernicke's area

Midline

Damage to Wernicke's area **Receptive dysphasia**

Primary auditory cortex

● Tonotopic organization
● Columns defined by:-
  callosal connection
  input from two ears

● Primary auditory area ≡ Brodmann area 41
● Secondary auditory area ≡ Brodmann area 41,42

Medial geniculate nucleus

Inferior colliculus → Superior colliculus

Nucleus of lateral lemniscus (NLL) — Probst's commissure — Nucleus of lateral lemniscus (NLL)

Lateral lemniscus

Superior olivary complex

Superior olivary complex

| Medial EE Low frequency | Lateral EI High frequency |

First site of binaural inputs

Frequency tuning

Superior olivary complex

Midline

Sound localization

Cochlear nucleus

Cochlea ← Ventral

Trapezoid body

E = Excitatory input from one ear
I = Inhibitory input from one ear

VIIIth cranial

Dorsal

Dorsal acoustic striae

Sounds <1400 Hz are detected by Δt but if frequency is >1400 Hz then wavelength of sound is less than distance between ears so phase or time difference is ambiguous—rely on ΔI

Amplitude

Log. frequency

Each fibre of auditory nerve has a characteristic frequency which is derived from hair cells at particular site on basilar membrane

Input from right cochlea   Input from left cochlea

A
B
C
D

Output

Azimuth

Angle of elevation

Possible arrangement to code for time differences in sound localization in superior olivary complex (SOC). Each SOC neurone is maximally activated by an input from each ear arriving at the same time at its axon hillock—the Δt component is coded for by the position of the synapses from each cochlea relative to this part of the neurone. Alternatively the coding can be done using different afferent axon lengths from each cochlear nucleus.

Head creates a delay Δt (i.e. time difference) in the sound reaching each ear and a reduction in intensity (ΔI) as head absorbs some of sound energy.
Pinna is critically important in localization of sound in the vertical plane.

The **vestibulocochlear or eighth cranial nerve** transmits information from both the cochlea and vestibular apparatus; the latter is discussed in Chapter 28. Each fibre of the cochlear nerve is selectively tuned to a characteristic frequency, which is determined by its site of origin within the cochlea (see Chapter 26). These fibres are then arranged according to the location of their innervating hair cells along the basilar membrane (BM), and this tonotopic organization is maintained throughout the auditory pathway.

On entering the brainstem the cochlear nerve synapses in the cochlear nuclear complex of the medulla.

Auditory pathways

The **cochlear nucleus** is divided into a ventral (VCN) and dorsal (DCN) part. The VCN projects to the superior olivary complex (SOC) bilaterally while the DCN projects via the dorsal acoustic striae to the contralateral nucleus of the lateral lemniscus and inferior colliculus.

The **SOC** contains spindle-shaped neurones with a lateral and medial dendrite, which receive an input from each ear. It is the first site of binaural interactions and so this structure is important in sound localization. In the **medial part of the SOC** this input is excitatory from each ear (**EE cells**) whereas in the **lateral SOC** the neurones have an excitatory input from one ear and an inhibitory input from the other (**EI cells**).

The EE cells by virtue of their input are important in the localization of sounds of low frequency (less than 1.4 kHz) where the critical factor is the delay (Δt) in the sound reaching one and then the other ear. One possible arrangement that could be employed is shown in the figure and relies on the differential localization of the synaptic inputs to a single SOC neurone from the two ears.

The EI cells are important in the localization of higher frequency sounds where the difference in intensity (ΔI) of sound between the two ears is important (ΔI being generated as a result of the head acting as a shield). Sounds of frequencies greater than 1.4 kHz (in the case of humans) rely on ΔI for localization. In the case of sounds originating in the midline, there will be no Δt and no ΔI and there is some confusion in localization which can be overcome to some extent by moving the head or using other sensory cues.

The localization of sound within the vertical plane is dependent in some way on the pinna.

The SOC not only projects rostrally to the **inferior colliculus (IC)** but also has an important input to the cochlea where it primarily con-

trols the OHCs and by so doing the response properties of the organ of Corti (see Chapter 26). The projection to the IC is tonotopic and this structure also receives an input from the primary auditory cortex (A1) and other sensory modalities. In this respect it interacts with the superior colliculus and is involved in the orienting response to novel audiovisual stimuli (see Chapters 24 and 40).

The IC projects to the **medial geniculate nucleus of the thalamus (MGN)**, which projects to the **A1** in the superior temporal gyrus. This area corresponds to Brodmann's areas 41 and 42, with the thalamic afferent input synapsing in layers III and IV of the cortex. The columnar organization of A1 is poorly defined but the tonotopic map is maintained so that low-frequency sounds are located posteriorly and high-frequency sounds anteriorly.

Secondary auditory cortical areas and language

In A1, apart from neurones with relatively simple afferent inputs, there are some cells that respond to complex sounds. These neurones are more frequently found in the **secondary auditory areas**, and reach their most complex in humans in **Wernicke's area**, the cortical site of language comprehension. This area is found in the dominant hemisphere (usually left) and when damaged (e.g. in cerebrovascular accidents (CVAs); see Chapter 17) leads to a *receptive* or *fluent dysphasia*, or an inability to understand what is being said. This area is connected, via the **arcuate fasciculus**, to an area in the dominant hemisphere frontal lobe known as **Broca's area**. This frontal area is responsible for the expression of speech and damage to it causes an *expressive* or *nonfluent dysphasia* which is an inability to speak fluently in the absence of damage to the motor apparatus of articulation. *Aphasia* is an inability to generate any speech and in a large middle cerebral artery CVA of the dominant hemisphere this can occur as both Wernicke's and Broca's areas are involved. Selective lesions of the arcuate fasciculus are said to produce a *conduction aphasia*, where the patient understands and can speak but cannot repeat words and sentences. However, current evidence points to a more complex interaction among brain regions in the recognition and production of speech.

Aphasia and dysphasia are to be distinguished from deficits in the activation and execution of the motor acts of speaking (e.g. weakness of the palate and tongue in *motorneurone disease*), which is termed *dysarthria* (or anarthria when no speech can be generated).

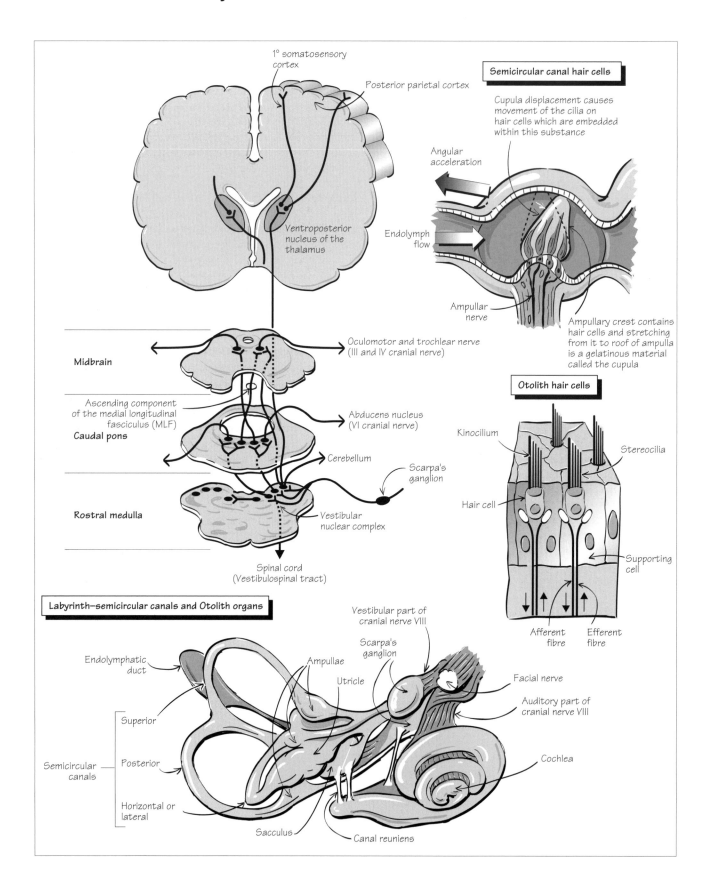

1° somatosensory cortex

Posterior parietal cortex

Ventroposterior nucleus of the thalamus

Semicircular canal hair cells

Cupula displacement causes movement of the cilia on hair cells which are embedded within this substance

Angular acceleration

Endolymph flow

Ampullar nerve

Ampullary crest contains hair cells and stretching from it to roof of ampulla is a gelatinous material called the cupula

Midbrain

Oculomotor and trochlear nerve (III and IV cranial nerve)

Ascending component of the medial longitudinal fasciculus (MLF)
Caudal pons

Abducens nucleus (VI cranial nerve)

Cerebellum

Scarpa's ganglion

Rostral medulla

Vestibular nuclear complex

Spinal cord (Vestibulospinal tract)

Otolith hair cells

Kinocilium

Stereocilia

Hair cell

Supporting cell

Afferent fibre

Efferent fibre

Labyrinth–semicircular canals and Otolith organs

Endolymphatic duct

Ampullae

Vestibular part of cranial nerve VIII

Scarpa's ganglion

Utricle

Facial nerve

Auditory part of cranial nerve VIII

Superior

Semicircular canals

Posterior

Horizontal or lateral

Cochlea

Sacculus

Canal reuniens

The vestibular system is concerned with balance, postural reflexes and eye movements. It consists of a peripheral transducer component which projects to the brainstem (including the oculomotor nuclei), and from there to the thalamus and sensory cortex as well as to the cerebellum and spinal cord. Disruption to the system results in the symptoms of dizziness, vertigo, nausea ± blurred vision with signs of eye movement abnormalities (typically nystagmus; see Chapter 40) and unsteadiness. In the comatose patient, clinical testing of the vestibular system can provide useful information on the integrity of the brainstem.

Vestibular transduction

The peripheral transducer component consists of the **labyrinth**, which is made up of two **otolith organs** (the **utricle** and the **sacculus**) together with the **ampullae** located in the three **semicircular canals**. The otolith organs are primarily concerned with static head position and linear acceleration while the semicircular canals are more concerned with rotational (angular) acceleration of the head.

Hair cells are found both in the otolith organs and the ampullae and are similar in structure to those found in the cochlea (see Chapters 19 and 26). As in the cochlea, deflection of the stereocilia towards the kinocilium depolarizes the cell and allows transmitter to be released from the hair cell, leading to activation of the associated afferent fibre. The converse is true if the stereocilia are deflected in the opposite direction. Movement of the cilia is associated with rotational movement of the head (ampullae receptors in the semicircular canals) and acceleration or tilting of the head (otolith organs in utricle), as although head movement causes the **endolymph** bathing the hair cells to move, it 'lags behind' and so distorts the stereocilia.

Spontaneous activity in the afferent fibres is high, reflecting the spontaneous leakage of transmitter from the cell at the synapse. Hyperpolarization of the hair cell therefore results in a reduced afferent discharge, while depolarization is associated with an increase in firing. Efferent fibres from the brainstem terminating on the hair cells can change the sensitivity of the receptor end-organ.

Peripheral disorders of the vestibular system

Damage to the peripheral vestibular system is not uncommon. An example of such a disorder is *benign positional vertigo* which commonly occurs after trauma or infection of the vestibular apparatus with the deposition of debris (e.g. otolith crystals or otoconia) typically in the posterior semicircular canal. This condition, which is characterized by paroxysms of vertigo, nausea and ataxia induced by turning the head into certain positions—such as lying down or rolling over in bed—is therefore the consequence of distortion of endolymph flow in this canal

secondary to the debris. Treatment and cure can be effected if a series of head manoeuvres are followed which allows the debris to fall out of the semicircular canal and into the ampullae. Viral infections of the vestibular apparatus are common (labyrinthitis) and can be severely disabling with profound dizziness and vomiting without any head movement. Such infections are usually self-limiting.

Bilateral failure of the vestibular apparatus can result in **oscillopsia**, a symptom describing an inability to visually fixate on objects especially with head movements (see Chapter 40). In contrast, powerful excitation of the vestibular system such as that encountered during motion sickness produces dizziness, vomiting, sweating and tachycardia, caused by discrepancies between vestibular and visual information.

Vestibular function can be tested by introducing water into the external meatus **(caloric testing)**. When warm water is applied to a seated subject whose head is tilted back by about 60°, nystagmus towards the treated side is observed. Cold water produces nystagmus towards the opposite side. These effects reflect the changes in the temperature of the endolymph and an effect resembling head rotation away from the irrigated side.

Central vestibular system and vestibular reflexes

Afferent vestibular fibres in the eighth cranial nerve have their cell bodies in the vestibular **(Scarpa's) ganglion** and terminate in one of the **four vestibular nuclei** in the medulla which also receive inputs from neck muscle receptors and the visual system.

The vestibular nuclei project to the spinal cord (see Chapters 12, 32 and 34), contralateral vestibular nuclei, the cerebellum and oculomotor nuclei, and the ipsi- and contralateral thalamus. Some of these structures are important in reflex eye movements such as the ability to maintain visual fixation while moving the head—the vestibulo-ocular reflex (VOR; see Chapters 40 and 47). Other projections of the vestibular nuclei are important in maintaining posture and gait. The cortical termination of the vestibular input to the central nervous system (CNS) is the primary somatosensory cortex (SmI) and the posterior parietal cortex (see Chapter 30).

Caloric testing of the vestibular system examines the integrity of the vestibular apparatus and its brainstem connections so it can be useful in comatosed patients when the degree of brainstem function needs to be ascertained. Less severe central damage to the vestibular apparatus can occur in a number of conditions including *multiple sclerosis* (see Chapter 54) and vascular insults (see Chapter 17). In most cases other structures are involved and so there are other symptoms and signs on examination.

29 Olfaction and taste

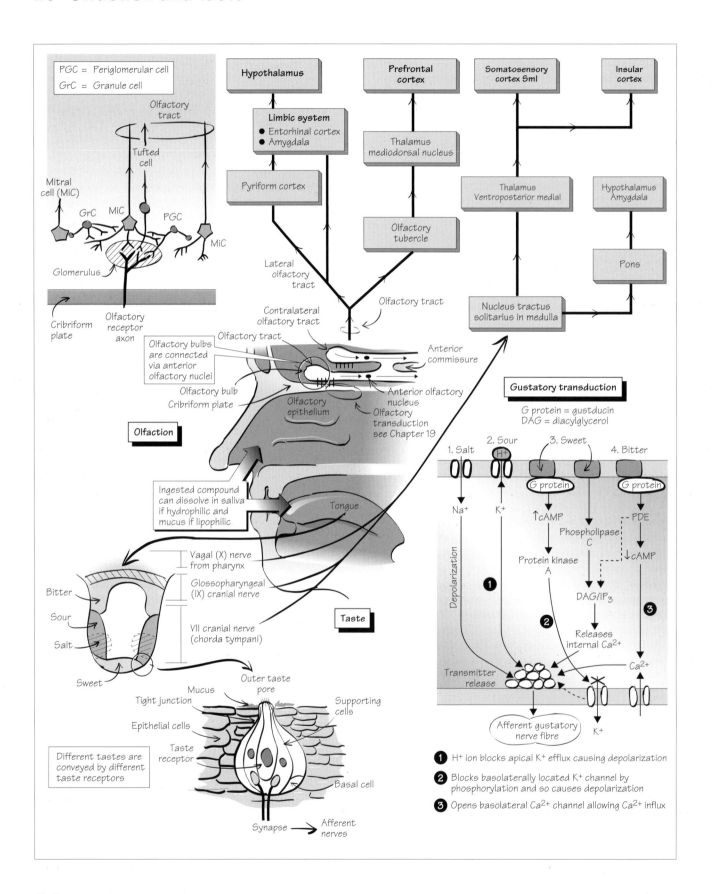

PGC = Periglomerular cell
GrC = Granule cell

Olfactory tract
Tufted cell
Mitral cell (MiC)
GrC   MiC   PGC
MiC
Glomerulus
Cribriform plate
Olfactory receptor axon

Hypothalamus

Limbic system
● Entorhinal cortex
● Amygdala

Pyriform cortex

Lateral olfactory tract

Contralateral olfactory tract

Prefrontal cortex

Thalamus mediodorsal nucleus

Olfactory tubercle

Olfactory tract

Somatosensory cortex SmI

Thalamus Ventroposterior medial

Insular cortex

Hypothalamus Amygdala

Pons

Nucleus tractus solitarius in medulla

Olfactory bulbs are connected via anterior olfactory nuclei
Olfactory tract
Olfactory bulb
Cribriform plate
Olfactory epithelium
Anterior commissure
Anterior olfactory nucleus
Olfactory transduction see Chapter 19

Olfaction

Ingested compound can dissolve in saliva if hydrophilic and mucus if lipophilic

Tongue

Vagal (X) nerve from pharynx
Glossopharyngeal (IX) cranial nerve
VII cranial nerve (chorda tympani)

Bitter
Sour
Salt
Sweet

Taste

Mucus
Tight junction
Epithelial cells
Taste receptor
Outer taste pore
Supporting cells
Basal cell
Synapse → Afferent nerves

Different tastes are conveyed by different taste receptors

Gustatory transduction

G protein = gustducin
DAG = diacylglycerol

1. Salt   2. Sour   3. Sweet   4. Bitter

G protein   G protein

Na$^+$ K$^+$ ↑cAMP   PDE

Phospholipase C   ↓cAMP

Protein kinase A

DAG/IP$_3$

Releases internal Ca^{2+}

Ca^{2+}

Depolarization

Transmitter release   K$^+$

Afferent gustatory nerve fibre

❶ H$^+$ ion blocks apical K$^+$ efflux causing depolarization

❷ Blocks basolaterally located K$^+$ channel by phosphorylation and so causes depolarization

❸ Opens basolateral Ca^{2+} channel allowing Ca^{2+} influx

The **olfactory or first cranial nerve** contains more fibres than any other sensory nerve projecting to the central nervous system (CNS), while **taste** is relayed via the seventh, ninth and tenth cranial nerves (see Chapter 14).

Olfaction

The olfactory system as a whole is able to discriminate a great diversity of different chemical stimuli or odours, and this is made possible through thousands of different olfactory receptors. These receptors are located in the apical dendrite of the olfactory receptor cell and the axon of this cell projects directly into the CNS via the cribriform plate at the top of the nose to the olfactory bulb.

The **olfactory stimulus or odour**, on binding to the olfactory receptor, depolarizes it (see Chapter 19) which, if sufficient, leads to the generation of action potentials at the cell body which are then conducted down the olfactory nerve axons to the olfactory bulb.

The **olfactory nerve** passes through the roof of the nose through a bone known as the cribriform plate. Damage to this structure (e.g. head trauma) can shear the olfactory nerve axons causing a loss of smell or *anosmia*. However, the most common cause of a loss of smell is local trouble within the nose, usually infection and inflammation. The olfactory receptor axons then synapse in the olfactory bulb that lies at the base of the frontal lobe. Damage to this structure, as occurs in frontal *meningiomas*, produces anosmia that can be unilateral.

The **olfactory bulb** contains a complex arrangement of cells. The axons from the olfactory nerve synapse on the apical dendrites of mitral and, to a lesser extent, tufted cells, both of which project out of the olfactory bulb as the olfactory tract. The olfactory bulb contains a number of inhibitory interneurones (granule and periglomerular cells) which are important in modifying the flow of olfactory information through the bulb.

The **olfactory tract** projects to the temporal lobe where it synapses in the **pyriform cortex** and **limbic system**, which projects to the **hypothalamus**. This projection is important in the behavioural effects of olfaction, which are perhaps more evident in other species. In humans, lesions in these structures rarely produce a pure anosmia, but activation of this area of the CNS as occurs in *temporal lobe epilepsy* (see Chapter 53) is associated with the abnormal perception of smells (e.g. olfactory hallucinations).

The projection of the olfactory system to the thalamus is small and is via the olfactory tubercle to the mediodorsal nucleus, which projects to the prefrontal cortex. The role of this pathway is not clear.

Taste

The **taste** or **gustatory receptors** are located in the tongue. They are clustered together in fungiform papillae with support and stem cells; the latter dividing to replace those gustatory receptors that are damaged. The apical surface of the gustatory receptor contains microvilli covered in mucus, which is generated by the neighbouring goblet cells. Any ingested compound can therefore reach the gustatory receptor; hydrophilic substances are dissolved in saliva while lipophilic substances are dissolved in the mucus. Taste is traditionally classified according to four modalities—salt, sour, sweet and bitter—which correlate well with the different transduction processes that are now known to exist for these different tastes. A fifth taste (uami) has also recently been described.

Salt stimuli cause a direct depolarization of the gustatory receptors by virtue of the fact that Na^+ passes through an amiloride-sensitive apical membrane channel. The depolarization leads to the release of neurotransmitter from the basal part of the cell which activates the afferent fibres in the relevant cranial nerve. **Sour stimuli**, in contrast, probably achieve a similar effect by the blocking of apical voltage-dependent H^+ channels. **Sweet stimuli** bind to a receptor that activates the G protein, gustducin, which then activates an adenylate cyclase with cyclic adenosine monophosphate (cAMP) production. The rise in cAMP activates a protein kinase that phosphorylates and closes basolateral K^+ channels and by so doing depolarizes the receptor. **Bitter stimuli** similarly rely on receptor binding and G-protein activation. One pathway involves gustducin but, in this instance, this leads to activation of a cAMP phosphodiesterase that reduces the level of cAMP (and so the phosphorylating protein kinase) leading to opening of the basolateral Ca^{2+} channels and so transmitter release. An alternative pathway for both sweet and bitter tastes involves the activation of a phospholipase C and the production of inositol triphosphate (IP_3) and diacylglycerol (DAG) which can release Ca^{2+} from internal stores within the receptor. The increased Ca^{2+} concentration promotes neurotransmitter release.

The receptors relay their information via the **chorda tympani** (anterior two-thirds of the tongue) and **glossopharyngeal nerve** (posterior third of the tongue) to **the nucleus of the solitary tract** in the medulla (see Chapters 13 and 14). The structure projects rostrally via the thalamus to the primary somatosensory cortex (SmI) and the insular cortex, with a possible further projection to the hypothalamus and amygdala. Some patients with *temporal lobe epilepsy* have an aura of an abnormal taste in the mouth which may be consequent of this latter projection (see Chapter 53).

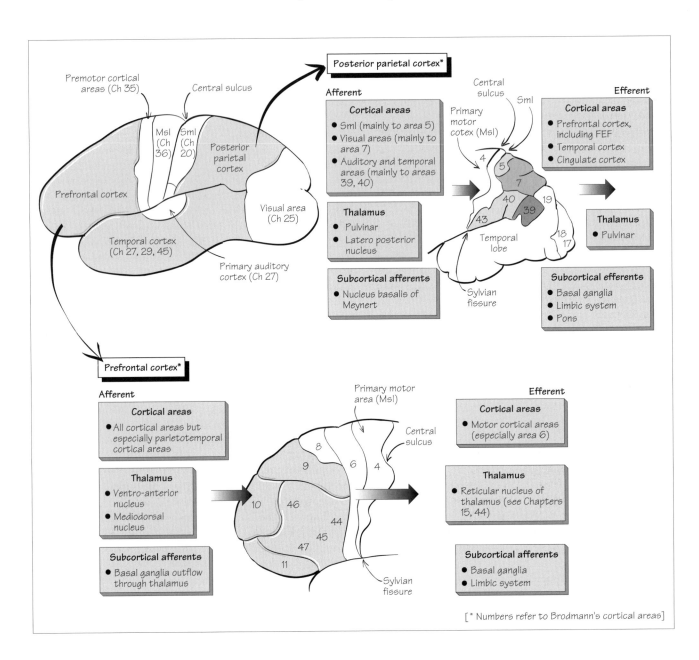

[* Numbers refer to Brodmann's cortical areas]

The **association cortices** are those parts of the cerebral cortex that do not have a primary motor or sensory role, but instead are involved in the higher order processing of sensory information necessary for perception and movement initiation.

These association areas include the posterior parietal cortex (PPC) (defined in monkeys as corresponding to Brodmann's areas 5 and 7, and in humans including areas 39 and 40); the prefrontal cortex (corresponding to Brodmann's areas 9–12 and 44–47) and the temporal cortex (corresponding to Brodmann's areas 21, 22, 37 and 41–43). The temporal cortex is involved in audition and language, complex visual processing (such as face recognition) and memory and is discussed in Chapters 25, 27 and 45.

Posterior parietal cortex

This area has developed greatly during evolution and is related to specific forms of human behaviour, such as the extensive use of tools, collaborative strategic planning and the development of language. It has two main subdivisions within it: one involved mainly with somatosensory information (centred on area 5); and the other with visual stimuli (centred on area 7).

Neurophysiologically, **area 5** contains many units with a complex sensory input often with a convergence of different sensory modalities, such as proprioceptive and cutaneous stimuli. These units with such a dual input are probably involved in the sensory control of posture and movements. Other units with multiple cutaneous inputs are probably more involved in object recognition. However, in addition to having these complex sensory inputs, units in this area are often only maximally activated when the sensory stimulus is of interest or behavioural significance. Damage to this area produces a contralateral sensory loss that is often subtle, e.g. a failure to recognize objects on tactile manipulation *(astereognosis)*. In addition, patients often demonstrate an inattention to stimuli received on the contralateral side of the body. This can be so severe that the patient denies the existence of that part of his or her body which can then interfere with the actions of the normal non-neglected side (intermanual conflict or alien limb). More commonly, the patient fails to perceive sensory stimuli contralaterally when stimuli are simultaneously applied to both sides of the body (extinction).

In contrast, **area 7** is more involved in complex visual processing, with many of the units in this area responding to stimuli of interest or behavioural significance (e.g. food). Many different units are found in this cortical area some of which maximally respond to the visual fixation and tracking, while others are more involved in the process of switching attention from one visual object of interest to another (light sensitive or visual space neurones). There are individual neurones in area 7 that respond to both sensory and visual stimuli. Some of these neurones are maximally activated when a stimulus is moved towards the neurone's cutaneous receptive field from extrapersonal (distant) space, while others are maximally activated during visual fixation of a desired object in which there is concomitant movement of the arm towards that object. In humans, damage to this area produces a neglect of visual stimuli in the contralateral hemifield, as well as defects in eye movement and the visual control of movement. However, a more striking deficit which may occur in some patients is in the realm of complex visual processing such as route finding and the construction of complex shapes.

Finally, in humans, and to a lesser extent in other primates and animals, units are found in the posterior parietal cortex that are maximally activated by vestibular and auditory inputs (see Chapters 27 and 28). Therefore damage to this area in humans can lead to complex difficulties in vision and visually guided movements, balance and language processing, including arithmetic skills. This includes an inability to write *(agraphia)*, to read *(alexia)* and calculate simple sums *(acalculia)*.

Prefrontal cortex

This cortical area has increased in size with phylogenetic development and has its greatest representation in humans. It is involved in the purposive behaviour of an organism and thus is intimately involved in the planning of responses to stimuli that include a motor component (see Chapter 32). Within this structure are specialized cortical areas such as the frontal eye fields (FEF; see Chapter 40) and Broca's area (see Chapter 27). Although the prefrontal cortex is treated as a functional whole this is a gross simplification.

Many different types of units are encountered neurophysiologically in this area of cortex, but they generally respond to complex sensory stimuli of behaviourial relevance, which can then be translated into a cue for movement.

Damage to this site in animals leads to increased distractability with corresponding deficits in working memory (the ability to retain information for more than a few seconds) and a change in locomotor activity and emotional responsiveness. A patient with frontal lobe damage anterior to the motor areas has a characteristic syndrome without insight. The patient is often disinhibited, which results in him or her behaving in an atypical, often childish, fashion. The patient has very poor attention and is easily distractable, cannot retain information and is sometimes unable to form new memories, with a tendency to perseverate (the repetition of words or phrases and actions) and pursue old patterns of behaviour even in the face of environmental change. He or she is unable to formulate and pursue goals and plans, to generalize and deduce. There is often a marked reduction in verbal output, which is also reflected in motor behaviour as evidenced by a lack of spontaneous movement with a change in food preference, typically favouring sweet over savoury foods. The patient can become apathetic with severe blunting of his or her emotional responses, although in some cases the converse is true with the patient becoming aggressive. Overall, the patient's personality changes and it is typically others who bring the patient to medical attention, as the patient usually denies there is any problem (no insight).

The reliance on the clinical symptomatology to describe the function of the prefrontal cortex relates to the fact that this part of the cortex is most developed in humans. However, extensive damage of the frontal lobes can also affect the cortical motor areas (see Chapter 35), eye movements (see Chapter 40), the ability to talk (an expressive dysphasia; see Chapter 27) and the control of micturition.

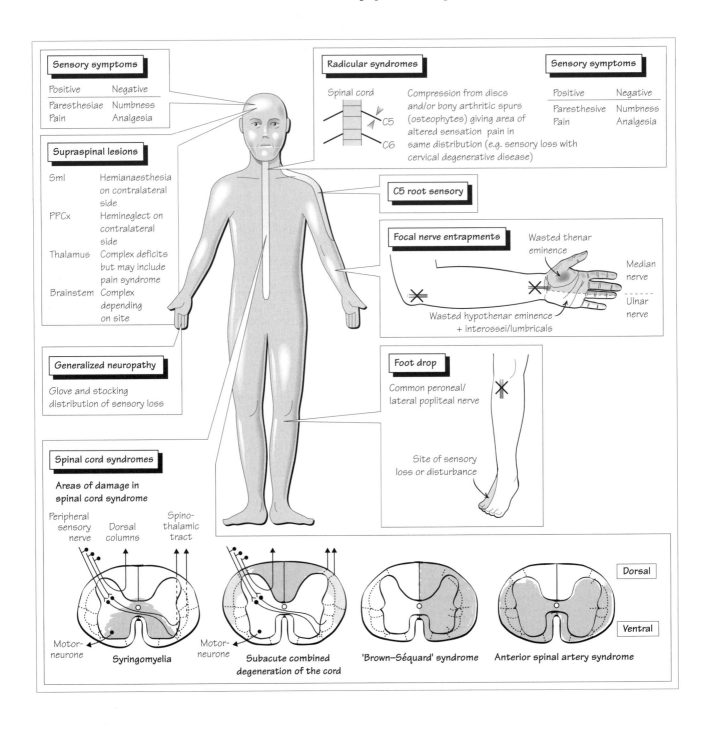

Disturbances in the sensory pathways can produce one of two main symptoms: negative ones, with a loss of sensation such as numbness or analgesia; or positive ones, such as pins and needles (paresthesiae) or pain. These symptoms can arise from many different sites along the sensory pathways, but it is often the distribution of sensory change that points towards the likely site of pathology.

In order to determine the nature and cause of the sensory disturbance a full history and examination is needed along with appropriate tests.

Most patients with isolated sensory symptoms do not yield to a diagnosis but the most common causes are probably neuropathies and multiple sclerosis.

A typical screen of tests for patients with sensory symptoms involves blood tests, nerve conduction studies (NCS) and magnetic resonance imaging (MRI) of brain and spinal cord. In all cases it is important to remember that non-neurological causes, e.g. hyperventilation, will give positive sensory symptoms, typically in the fingers and peri-orally.

Peripheral nerve

Diseases of the peripheral nerves can cause sensory disturbance. This can either be caused by *focal nerve entrapment* or *a generalized neuropathy*, in which case the disease process can either target the large or small fibres.

Common focal nerve entrapments include:
• The median nerve at the wrist (*carpel tunnel syndrome*). Patients typically present with aching in the forearm, weakness of some of the thumb muscles and loss of sensation over the thumb and adjacent two and half fingers. It often resolves spontaneously but in cases where it does not, a simple surgical decompression is often curative.
• The ulnar nerve at the elbow. Patients present with wasting of most of the intrinsic hand muscles with weakness and loss of sensation in the hand involving the little and half of the ring finger but without involvement of the forearm. It can be treated by surgical transposition of the nerve in some cases.
• The common peroneal (or lateral popliteal nerve) can be trapped around the knee. Patients typically present with foot drop and numbness on the outer aspect of the foot.

Generalized neuropathies are the result of many causes and if large fibres are involved then there is a loss of joint position sense, vibration perception and light touch along with the loss of reflexes. These neuropathies are rarely purely sensory in nature so are often associated with weakness and wasting. The typical pattern of sensory loss in these neuropathies is 'glove and stocking' which, as the name implies, reflects the loss of sensation to the forearm and to the shin/knee.

In some cases patients complain of much pain but paradoxically have reduced sensation for pain and temperature. These patients are more likely to have a *small fibre neuropathy*.

Rarely, the dorsal root ganglion cell (as opposed to the peripheral nerve) is targeted by the disease process. In these instances there is a devastating loss of proprioception.

Peripheral pain syndromes are discussed in Chapters 21 and 22, but it is always important to remember that pain is more often the result of non-neurological causes such as arthritis or local tissue damage.

The nerves as they emerge out of the spinal column can be trapped typically by bony spurs or intravertebral discs and give sensory disturbance along that nerve root. Patients normally complain of pain radiating down that nerve root with sensory abnormalities confined to that dermatome (see Chapter 1). This commonly happens in the cervical and lumbar region and may require surgical decompression. In such cases there is weakness, wasting and loss of the appropriate reflexes.

Spinal cord

The different courses of the spinal pathways for sensation can lead to distinctive syndromes.

Syringomyelia

Syringomyelia is the development, for a number of reasons, of a cyst or cavity around or near to the central canal, usually in the cervical region. The lesion typically disrupts the spinothalamic tract (STT) fibres as they cross just ventral to the central canal, resulting in a dissociated sensory loss, i.e. reduced temperature and pain sensation at the level of the lesion but normal light touch, vibration perception and joint position sense (see Chapter 20). In addition there may be motor involvement because of expansion of the cyst into the ventral horn or laterally into the descending motor tracts.

Subacute combined degeneration of the spinal cord

This is usually associated with pernicious anaemia and a lack of vitamin B_{12}. It is characterized by demyelination and eventually degeneration of the dorsal columns (DCs), the spinocerebellar tracts and the corticospinal tract (CoST) and in addition there is damage to peripheral nerves (*peripheral neuropathy*). Patients therefore develop a combination of paraesthesiae and sensory loss (especially light touch, vibration perception and joint position sense) with weakness and incoordination (see Chapter 20).

Brown–Séquard syndrome

This describes a lesion involving one half of the cord such that there is an ipsilateral loss of position and tactile senses (DC sensory information), a contralateral loss of temperature sensation originating from several segments below the lesion (STT sensory information), and ipsilateral spasticity and weakness because of involvement of the CoST pathway (see Chapters 21 and 22).

Anterior spinal artery syndrome

This syndrome describes the situation when there is occlusion of the artery providing blood to the anterior two-thirds of the cord. The patient has weakness and sensory loss to temperature and pain with preservation of DC sensory modalities such as joint position sense and vibration perception (see Chapter 17).

Transverse myelitis

Transverse myelitis (not shown in figure) describes a complete lesion of the whole spinal cord at one level which produces a complete sensory loss with weakness from that level down. The weakness is characteristically caused by a disruption of both the descending motor pathways and the spinal motorneurones. It is typically seen as a part of *multiple sclerosis* or a secondary acute demyelinating process in response to some infection such as an atypical pneumonia.

Brain

Abnormalities in supraspinal sites can result from a variety of causes and depending on the disease process and site determines the type of sensory disturbance. Typically, hemispheric lesions give a loss of sensation down the contralateral side of the body. Brainstem lesions give a range of sensory deficits depending on the exact level of the lesion; thus, pontine lesion can give ipsilateral sensory loss of the face but contralateral sensory loss in the limbs.

Cortical lesions can give a loss of sensation if the primary somatosensory cortex is involved, or can give more complex sensory deficits such as astereognosis (an inability to recognize objects by touch) or even sensory neglect or inattention. These latter abnormalities are typically seen with lesions of the posterior parietal cortex.

In some cases, irritative lesions of the primary sensory cortex give rise to simple partial seizures (see Chapter 53) in which the patient experiences brief migrating sensory symptoms up one side of the body.

Pain syndromes can also develop with central lesions and this is best seen in small thalamic vascular events, where dysaesthesia is found in the contralateral limb in a typically diffuse distribution (see Chapter 22).

32 The organization of the motor systems

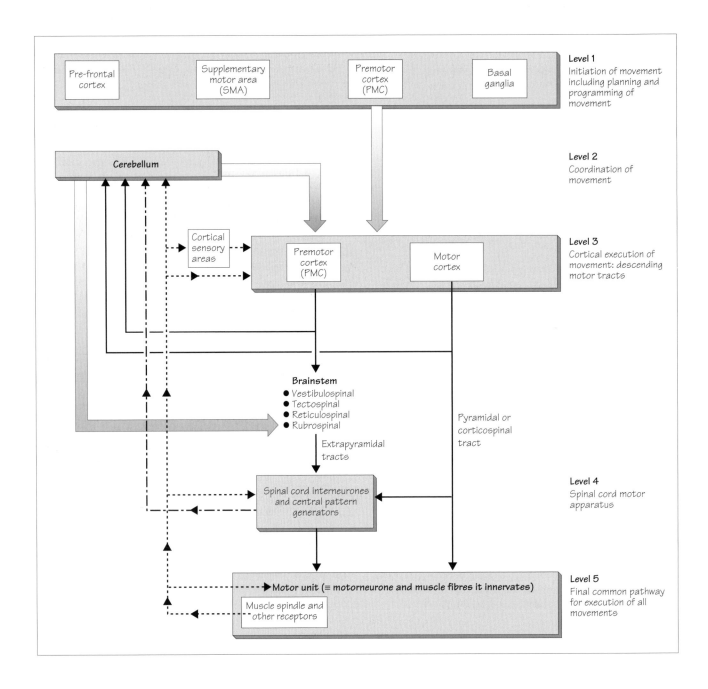

The **motor systems** are those areas of the nervous system that are primarily responsible for controlling movement. The movement can either be guided by inputs from the sensory systems (**closed-loop or reflexly controlled**) or triggered by a sensory cue or some internal desire to move (**open-loop or volitional movement**). In practice, most motor acts involve both types of movement, with closed-loop movements predominantly involving the axial or proximal muscles responsible for balance, posture and locomotion while the open-loop movements are typically associated with the distal musculature concerned with the control of fine skilled movements.

The organization of the motor structures is best viewed in terms of a hierarchy.

Level 1

The highest level of motor control is concerned with the **initiation, planning and programming of movements** in response to an internal desire to move. This desire probably originates in the **limbic system** (see Chapter 45) and **prefrontal** and **posterior parietal cortex** (see Chapter 30), while the structures primarily responsible for translating that desire into a movement are the **basal ganglia** (see Chapters 38 and 39) and their cortical projection areas in the frontal lobe (see Chapters 35 and 36). These cortical areas include the **supplementary motor area (SMA)** and **premotor cortex (PMC)**; the latter also has a specific role in the control of proximal muscles (see below).

Damage to the basal ganglia and their cortical projection sites leads to a range of complex movement disorders, which includes *Parkinson's disease*, as well as the development of abnormal involuntary movements such as *chorea*, *dystonia* and *ballismus* (see Chapter 39 for the definition of these terms). Damage to these areas does *not* produce any specific weakness or changes in the monosynaptic tendon reflexes (see Chapter 33).

Level 2

The next level is occupied by the **cerebellum**, which is responsible for the **coordination of movement**. It achieves this by comparing the intended movement descending from the motor areas in the cerebral cortex with the actual movement as detected by the activity of muscle afferents and interneurones (INs) in the spinal cord. It is capable of storing motor information, and this motor memory is not only useful in the learning of new movements but also in the correct timing of muscle activations during complex movements.

Damage to this structure leads primarily to a breakdown in the coordination of movement, without any specific weakness (see Chapter 37).

Level 3

The middle level is concerned with the control of the lower motorneurones (MNs) by the supraspinal **descending motor pathways**. This can broadly be divided into two sets of pathways.

1 The corticospinal (CoST) or pyramidal tract which originates in the motor, premotor and somatosensory cortices and synapses directly on to the MN in the brainstem cranial nerve nuclei and ventral (or anterior) horn of the spinal cord and to a lesser extent INs.

2 The extrapyramidal tracts which originate from subcortical structures and have a more complex distribution of synaptic contacts with both MNs and INs. These extrapyramidal pathways include the vestibulo- (VeST), reticulo- (ReST), tecto- (TeST) and rubrospinal tracts (RuST) and are all in receipt of an input from the primary motor cortex.

Damage in the central nervous system (CNS) is rarely specific to a single tract but interruption of the descending motor pathways produces a pattern of weakness in the limbs that is more pronounced in the extensor muscles in the arms and flexor muscles in the legs—the so-called (but misnamed) **pyramidal distribution of weakness**. In association with the weakness, there is increased tone in the muscles and brisk reflexes; all three features characterizing an *upper MN lesion* (see Chapter 41). In contrast to the higher levels in the hierarchy, this is the first level where damage is actually associated with weakness.

Level 4

A low level of motor organization is to be found in the **spinal cord** itself. The descending motor pathways from the brain synapse not only on the MNs, but also the INs and while some of these mediate the spinal cord **reflexes**, others are capable of generating their own outputs to MNs independently of any descending or peripheral sensory input—**central pattern generators**. These are important in locomotion (see Chapter 34).

Level 5

The lowest level or **final common pathway of the motor system** is the output neurone of the CNS to the muscle (the **MN**). The MN receives information not only from the brain via the descending pathways and spinal cord INs but also has an important input from sensory organs in the periphery, especially the **muscle spindle** and **Golgi tendon organ** that are found in the muscle and tendon, respectively (see Chapter 33). The muscle spindle in particular is important in mediating the **simple stretch reflex** that underlies the tendon jerks of the clinical examination.

Damage to the MN or its axon to the muscle produces a *lower* (as opposed to upper) *MN lesion*, characterized by weakness and wasting, hypotonia and reduced or absent reflexes (see Chapters 33 and 41).

A cautionary note

It is important to remember that the division of the CNS into motor and sensory functions is a gross simplification as all the motor areas have some sensory input. It is difficult to know the point at which a highly processed sensory input becomes the impulse for the initiation of a movement. It should also be realized that the division of the motor systems into various levels and different motor pools is a convenient but not strictly accurate device for understanding the control of movement and the pathophysiology of disorders of the motor system.

33 The muscle spindle and lower motorneurone

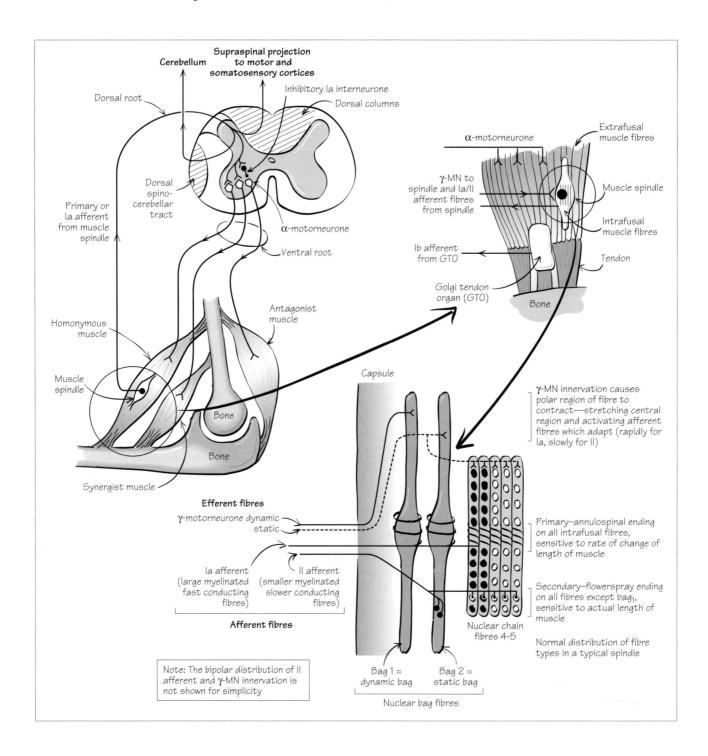

Lower motorneurone

The **lower motorneurone (LMN)** is defined as the neurone whose cell body lies in either the anterior or ventral horn of the spinal cord or cranial nerve nuclei of the brainstem and which directly innervates the muscle via its axon. The number of muscle fibres innervated by a single axon is termed the **motor unit**. The smaller the number of fibres per

motorneurone (MN) axon, the finer the control (e.g. the extraocular muscles).

The MNs of the anterior horn are divided into two types: the **α-MN** (70 μm in diameter) which innervate the muscle itself (the force generating extrafusal fibres); and the **γ-MN** (30 μm in diameter) which innervate the intrafusal fibres of the muscle spindle. The **muscle spindle** is an encapsulated sense organ found within the muscle, which is responsible for detecting the extent of muscle contraction by monitoring the length of muscle fibres.

It is the muscle spindle and its connections to the spinal cord that mediates the **tendon reflexes**; sudden stretching of a muscle by a sharp tap of a tendon hammer transiently activates the **Ia afferent nerve endings** which, via an excitatory monosynaptic input to the MN, causes that muscle (the **homonymous muscle**) to contract briefly (e.g. the knee jerk). In addition, the Ia afferent input from the muscle spindle, while activating other **synergistic muscles** with a similar action to the homonymous muscle, also inhibits muscles with opposing actions (**antagonist muscles**) through a **Ia inhibitory interneurone (IN)** in the spinal cord. However, it must be stressed that tendon jerks reflect not only the integrity of this circuit but the overall excitability of the MN, which is increased in cases of an upper MN lesion (see Chapter 41).

Muscle spindle

The **muscle spindle** lies in parallel to the extrafusal muscle fibres and consists of the following.
• **Nuclear bag and chain fibres** which have different morphological properties: the bag 1 or dynamic fibres are very sensitive to the rate of change in muscle length, while the bag 2 or static bag fibres are like the nuclear chain fibres in being more sensitive to the absolute length of the muscle.
• A γ-MN that synapses at the polar ends of the intrafusal muscle fibres and which can be one of two types: **dynamic or static**, with the latter innervating all but the bag 1 fibres. Both types of γ-MN are usually coactivated with the α-MN so that the intrafusal fibres contract at the same time as do the extrafusal fibres, thus ensuring that the spindle maintains its sensitivity during muscle contraction. Occasionally, the γ-MN can be activated independently of the α-MN, typically when the animal is learning some new complex movement, which increases the sensitivity of the spindle to changes in length.
• Two types of afferent fibres and nerve endings: a **Ia afferent fibre** associated with an annulospiral nerve ending winding around the centre of all types of intrafusal fibres (**primary ending**); and a slower conducting **type II fibre** which is associated with flowerspray endings on the more polar regions of the intrafusal fibres (with the exception of the bag 1 fibres; the **secondary ending**). The stretching of the intrafusal fibre activates both types of fibre. However, the Ia fibre is most sensitive to the rate of change in fibre length, while the type II fibres respond more to the overall length of the fibre rather than the rate of change in fibre length.

The spindle relays via the dorsal root to a number of central nervous system (CNS) sites including: (i) the MNs innervating the homonymous and synergistic muscles (the basis of the stretch reflex); (ii) INs inhibiting the antagonist muscles; (iii) the cerebellum via the dorsal spinocerebellar tract; (iv) the somatosensory cortex; and (v) the primary motor cortex via the dorsal column–medial lemniscal pathways. Thus, the muscle spindle is not only responsible for mediating simple stretch or tendon reflexes but is also involved in the coordination of movement, the perception of joint position (proprioception) and the modulation of long-latency or transcortical reflexes (see Chapter 36).

Damage to the spindle afferent fibres (e.g. in large fibre *neuropathies*) produces hypotonia (as the stretch reflex is important in controlling the normal tone of muscles), incoordination, reduced joint position sense and occasionally tremor with an inability to learn new motor skills in the face of novel environmental situations. In addition, large fibre neuropathies disrupt other somatosensory afferent inputs (see Chapters 20 and 31).

The **Golgi tendon organ** is found at the junction between muscle and tendon and thus lies in series with the extrafusal muscle fibres. It monitors the degree of muscle contraction in terms of the muscular force generated and relays this to the spinal cord via a **Ib afferent fibre**. This sensory organ, in addition to providing useful information to the CNS on the degree of tension within muscles, serves to prevent excessive muscular contractions (see Chapter 34).

Motorneurone recruitment and damage

The **'principle of recruitment'** corresponds to the order in which different types of muscle fibres are activated. The smallest α-MNs, which are those most easily excited by any input, innervate type 1 (*not* to be confused with the bag 1 intrafusal fibres found in the spindle) or slow-contracting fibres which are responsible for increasing and maintaining the tension in a muscle.

The next population of MNs to be activated are those that innervate the type 2A or fast-contracting/resistant to fatigue fibres which are responsible for virtually all forms of locomotion. Finally, the largest MNs are only activated by maximal inputs, which innervate type 2B or fast-contracting/easily fatigued fibres that are responsible for running or jumping.

The order of recruitment of MNs to a given input follows a simple relationship known as the **size principle**, which allows muscles to contract in a logical sequence.

The **α-MN itself can be damaged** in a number of different conditions but in all cases the clinical features are the same; there is wasting of the denervated muscles with weakness, and reduced or absent reflexes (a lower MN lesion).

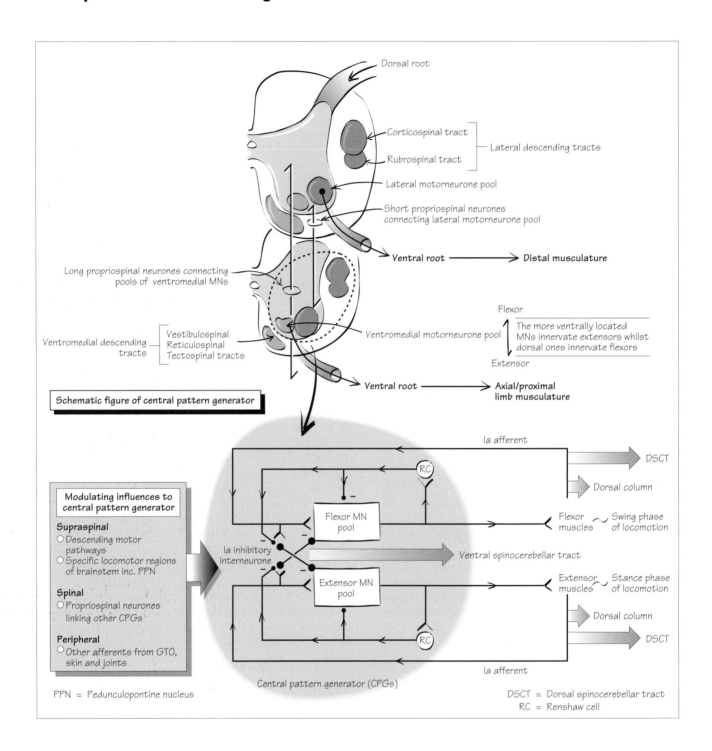

Schematic figure of central pattern generator

Dorsal root

Corticospinal tract — Lateral descending tracts

Rubrospinal tract

Lateral motorneurone pool

Short propriospinal neurones connecting lateral motorneurone pool

Ventral root ⟶ Distal musculature

Long propriospinal neurones connecting pools of ventromedial MNs

Flexor

The more ventrally located MNs innervate extensors whilst dorsal ones innervate flexors

Extensor

Ventromedial descending tracts — Vestibulospinal Reticulospinal Tectospinal tracts

Ventromedial motorneurone pool

Ventral root ⟶ Axial/proximal limb musculature

la afferent

DSCT

Dorsal column

RC

Flexor MN pool

Flexor muscles ⁓ Swing phase of locomotion

la inhibitory interneurone

Ventral spinocerebellar tract

Extensor MN pool

Extensor muscles ⁓ Stance phase of locomotion

Dorsal column

RC

DSCT

la afferent

Modulating influences to central pattern generator

Supraspinal
○ Descending motor pathways
○ Specific locomotor regions of brainstem inc. PPN

Spinal
○ Propriospinal neurones linking other CPGs

Peripheral
○ Other afferents from GTO, skin and joints

Central pattern generator (CPGs)

PPN = Pedunculopontine nucleus

DSCT = Dorsal spinocerebellar tract
RC = Renshaw cell

Spinal cord motor organization

In addition to containing the α- and γ-motorneurones (MNs), the spinal cord also contains a large number of **interneurones (INs)** which relay afferent information from the periphery and supraspinal sites. These INs can form networks which are intrinsically active and whose output governs the activity of MNs, **central pattern generators (CPGs)**. These CPGs, which may underlie locomotion, while not requiring any afferent input in order to produce a patterned motor output, are nevertheless modulated by both central and peripheral inputs (see Chapters 33 and 35).

Descending motor pathways (see Appendix 2b for details of individual tracts)

The **descending motor pathways** can be classified according to:

• their site of origin, namely pyramidal or extrapyramidal tracts (although *clinically* extrapyramidal disorders refer to diseases of the basal ganglia; see Chapter 39); or
• their location within the cord and the muscles they ultimately innervate through the MNs. Thus, the **pyramidal (corticospinal)** and **rubrospinal tract** are associated with a **lateral MN pool** that innervates the distal musculature, while the **vestibulo-, reticulo- and tectospinal tracts** are more associated with a **ventromedial MN pool** that innervates the axial and proximal musculature.

These latter MNs are linked by long **propriospinal neurones**, while the converse is true for the lateral MN pool. Thus, the **lateral motor system** is more involved in the control of fine distal movements, while the **ventromedial system** is more concerned with balance and posture.

The MNs of the anterior horn are further organized such that the most ventrally located MNs innervate the extensor muscles, while those found at more dorsal locations innervate the flexor musculature.

Locomotion

The control of **locomotion** is complex, as it requires the coordinated movement of all four limbs in most mammals.

Each cycle in locomotion is termed a **step** and involves a **stance** and a **swing** phase—the latter being that part of the cycle when the foot is not in contact with the ground. Each cycle requires the correct sequential activation of flexors and extensors. The simplest way to achieve this is to have **two CPGs (half centres)** that activate flexors and extensors, respectively, and which mutually inhibit each other.

This mutual inhibition can perhaps best be modelled using the **inhibitory Ia IN** and **Renshaw cells**. Renshaw cells are INs that, when activated by MNs, inhibit those same MNs (see Chapter 8). Thus, the activation of a MN pool by a CPG leads to its own inhibition and the removal of an inhibitory input to the antagonistic CPG, thus switching the muscle groups activated. This half centre model for locomotion can be modulated by a range of descending and peripheral inputs. In this latter respect the Ib afferent from the Golgi tendon organ (GTO) can switch the CPGs to prevent excessive tension developing in a muscle, while a range of cutaneous inputs can cause the cycle to be modified in the event of an obstacle being encountered. These afferents, termed **flexor reflex afferents**, cause the limb to be flexed so stepping over or withdrawing from the noxious or obstructive object.

CPGs within the spinal cord communicate with each other through propriospinal neurones. In contrast, supraspinal communication of information from and about the CPGs is relayed indirectly in the form of muscle spindle Ia afferent activity via the dorsal spinocerebellar tract (DSCT) and dorsal columns and spinal cord interneuronal activity via the ventral spinocerebellar tract (VSCT).

Clinical disorders of spinal cord motor control and locomotion

Although experimental animals can locomote in the absence of any significant supraspinal inputs (**fictive locomotion**), this is not the case in humans. However, clinical disorders of gait are relatively common and may occur for a number of reasons.

Disorders of spinal cord INs such as occurs in *stiff-person syndrome* are rare. In this condition the patient presents with increased tone or rigidity in the axial muscles ± spasms caused by the continuous firing of the MNs as a result of the loss of an inhibitory interneuronal input primarily to the ventromedial MNs. This condition is associated with antibodies against the synthetic enzyme for γ-aminobutyric acid (GABA), glutamic acid decarboxylase (GAD).

Damage to the descending pathways can produce a range of deficiencies. The most devastating is that seen with extensive brainstem damage when there is uninhibited extensor muscle activity and the patient adopts a characteristic *decerebrate posture* with arching of the neck and back and rigid extension of all four limbs. In contrast, a more rostrally placed lesion in one of the cerebral hemispheres produces weakness down the contralateral side (hemiplegia or hemiparesis) with increased tone (hypertonia) and increased tendon reflexes (hypereflexia) which may produce spontaneous or stretch-induced rhythmic involuntary muscular contractions (clonus). This situation is also seen with interruption of the descending motor pathways in the spinal cord (see Chapters 31, 32 and 41).

The pattern of weakness in such lesions characteristically involves the extensors more than the flexors in the upper limb and the converse in the lower limb. This is misleadingly termed a **pyramidal distribution of weakness**, as damage confined to the pyramidal tract in monkeys leads only to a deficiency in fine finger movements with a degree of hypotonia and hyporeflexia.

35 The cortical motor areas

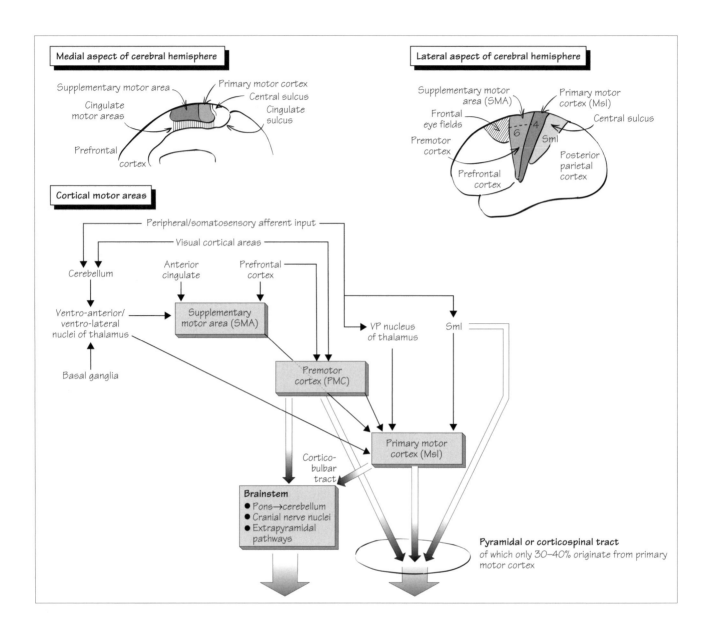

There are a number of cortical areas involved with the control of movement including the primary motor cortex (see Chapter 36), premotor cortex (PMC), supplementary motor area (SMA) and a number of adjacent areas in the anterior cingulate cortex. In addition, there are other areas that have specific roles in the cortical control of movement, including the frontal eye fields (see Chapter 40) and posterior parietal cortex (see Chapter 30). This chapter briefly discusses the organization of the motor cortical areas and their relative roles in movement control, while the next chapter concentrates on the primary motor cortex.

Primary motor cortex

The **primary motor cortex (MsI)** is that part of the cerebral cortex that produces a motor response with the minimum electrical stimulation. It corresponds to Brodmann's area 4 and lies just in front of the central sulcus and projects to the motorneurones (MNs) of the brainstem via the **corticobulbar tracts** and to the MNs of the spinal cord directly via the **corticospinal tract (CoST)** and indirectly via the subcortical extrapyramidal tracts. Indeed, MsI is particularly closely associated with the pyramidal tract (even though 60–70% of it originates in other cortical areas) and so has a role in the control of distal musculature and fine movements (see Chapters 34 and 36).

Other cortical areas

A range of other cortical areas are involved in the control of movement, including the **PMC** (corresponding to the lateral part of Brodmann's area 6); the **SMA** (corresponding to the medial aspect of Brodmann's area 6); a number of motor areas centred on the **anterior cingulate cortex** on the medial aspect of the frontal lobe; the **frontal eye fields** (corresponding to Brodmann's area 8) and the **posterior parietal cortex** (especially Brodmann's area 7).

Table 35.1 Cortical motor areas: connections and functions.

Cortical area	Afferent input	Efferent output	Neurophysiology	Function

Primary motor cortex (MsI)	SMA
	PMC
	SmI
	Cerebellum via thalamus (VA–VL nuclei)
	
	Dorsal column–medial lemniscal system (vp via nucleus of thalamus)
		Corticospinal or pyramidal tract
		Brainstem:
		  Pons to cerebellum
		  Cranial nerve nuclei
		  Extrapyramidal tracts
			Lesion of MsI results in a loss of placing, hopping reactions and skilled manipulative movements	Control of distal musculature and fine skilled movements
				Role in reflex control of movement (transcortical reflexes)

Premotor cortex (PMC)	SMA
	Prefrontal cortex
	Somatosensory and visual cortices
	Cerebellum via thalamus (VA–VL nuclei)
	Basal ganglia via thalamus (VA–VL nuclei)
		MsI
		Corticospinal or pyramidal tract
		Brainstem:
		  pons to cerebellum
		  extrapyramidal pathways
			Lesion of PMC produces a mild paresis and impairment of skilled movements; deficits in executing visuomotor tasks
			Regional blood flow studies show it is activated during tasks requiring directional guidance of a movement from sensory information
				Control of proximal musculature
				Control of movement sequence and preparation for movement

Supplementary motor area (SMA)	Prefrontal cortex Basal ganglia via thalamus (VA–VL nuclei) Anterior cingulate cortex Contralateral SMA	SMA (contralateral) PMC MsI	Lesion of SMA produces a severe reduction in spontaneous motor activity with forced grasping and failure of bimanual coordination Stimulation of SMA produces vocalization and complex bilateral arm movements Activity in SMA precedes any changes in MsI Units in SMA respond maximally to sensory cues being used as an instruction for a movement Regional blood-flow studies have shown an increased flow with the planning or thinking of a motor act	Role in the initiation and planning of movement Role in bimanual coordination

Some of these areas have specialist functions such as the frontal eye fields with eye movement control (see Chapter 40) and the posterior parietal cortex with the visual control of movement (see Chapter 30). The remaining areas in the frontal lobe are involved with more complex aspects of movement. Most of these other cortical areas therefore occupy a higher level in the motor hierarchy than MsI, and their connections and functions are summarized in the figure and Table 35.1 (see also Chapter 32).

The PMC refers to a specific area of Brodmann's area 6, and like the primary motor cortex has an input directly to the spinal MNs via the corticospinal or pyramidal tract. This area therefore occupies two levels of the motor hierarchy as it also has a role in the planning of movement (see Chapter 32). In contrast, the SMA lies medial to the PMC, has a much more clearly defined role in the planning of movements especially in response to sensory cues. Furthermore, it is now clear that the SMA is part of a much larger number of higher order motor cortical areas that lie along the medial side of the frontal cortex and which are involved in the planning of movements more than their execution. It is these cortical areas that receive the predominant outflow of the basal ganglia (see Chapter 38), and helps explain the abnormal movements that are seen with diseases of this area of the brain (see Chapter 39). For example, in *Parkinson's disease* there is a slowness and poverty of movement that is associated with underactivation of these cortical areas, a situation that is rectified by the administration of antiparkinsonian medication or successful neurosurgical interventions.

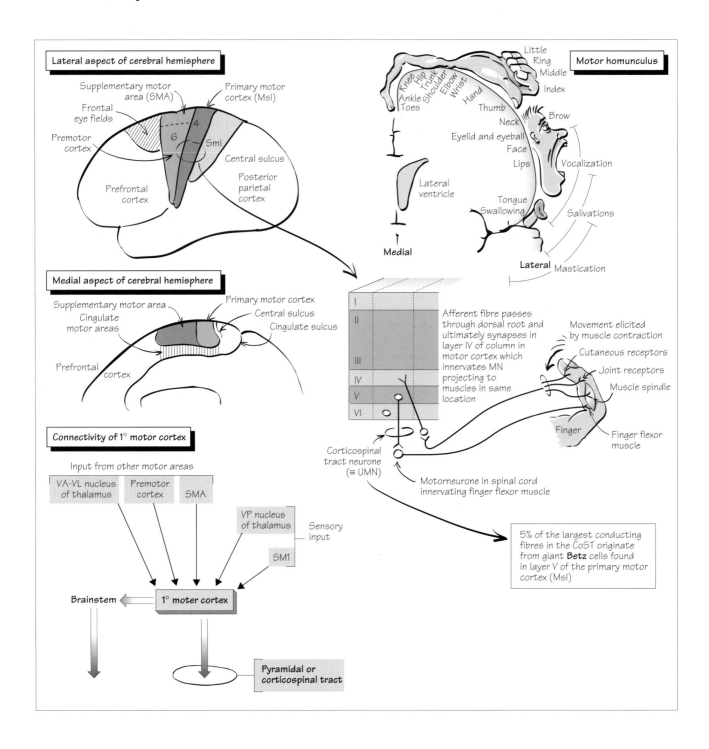

Lateral aspect of cerebral hemisphere

Supplementary motor area (SMA)
Frontal eye fields
Premotor cortex
Prefrontal cortex
Primary motor cortex (Msl)
Central sulcus
Posterior parietal cortex
4
6
Sml

Motor homunculus

Little
Ring
Middle
Index
Knee
Hip
Trunk
Shoulder
Elbow
Wrist
Hand
Ankle
Toes
Thumb
Neck
Brow
Eyelid and eyeball
Face
Lips
Vocalization
Lateral ventricle
Tongue
Swallowing
Salivations
Medial
Lateral
Mastication

Medial aspect of cerebral hemisphere

Supplementary motor area
Cingulate motor areas
Prefrontal cortex
Primary motor cortex
Central sulcus
Cingulate sulcus

I
II
III
IV
V
VI

Afferent fibre passes through dorsal root and ultimately synapses in layer IV of column in motor cortex which innervates MN projecting to muscles in same location

Movement elicited by muscle contraction
Cutaneous receptors
Joint receptors
Muscle spindle
Finger
Finger flexor muscle

Corticospinal tract neurone (≡ UMN)

Motorneurone in spinal cord innervating finger flexor muscle

5% of the largest conducting fibres in the CoST originate from giant **Betz** cells found in layer V of the primary motor cortex (Msl)

Connectivity of 1° motor cortex

Input from other motor areas

VA-VL nucleus of thalamus
Premotor cortex
SMA
VP nucleus of thalamus
Sensory input
SM1

Brainstem
1° motor cortex
Pyramidal or corticospinal tract

The primary motor cortex (MsI) receives afferent information from the cerebellum (via the thalamus), more anteriorly placed motor cortical areas such as the supplementary motor area (SMA) and a sensory input from the muscle spindle as well as cortical sensory areas. This latter sensory input emphasizes the artificial way in which the central nervous system (CNS) is divided up into motor and sensory systems and in order to acknowledge this the primary motor cortex is termed the MsI while the primary somatosensory cortex is termed the SmI (see Chapter 20).

Investigation of the **organization of MsI** has shown that the motor innervation of the body is organized in a highly topographical fashion, with the cortical representation of each body part being proportional to the degree of motor innervation — so, for example, the hand and orobuccal musculature have a large cortical representation. The resultant distorted image of the body in MsI is known as the **motor homunculus**, with the head represented laterally and the feet medially.

This organization may be manifest clinically in patients with *epilepsy* that originates in the motor cortex. In such cases the epileptic fit may begin at one site, typically the hand, and then spread so that the jerking marches out from the site of origin (**Jacksonian march**, named after the neurologist, Hughlings Jackson). This is in contrast to the clinical picture seen with seizures arising from the SMA, in which the patient raises both arms and vocalizes with complex repetitive movements suggesting that this area has a higher role in motor control (see Chapter 35).

These studies on the motor homunculus by Penfield and colleagues in the 1950s revealed the macroscopic organization of MsI, but subsequent microelectrode studies in animals revealed that MsI is composed of **cortical columns** (see Chapter 15). The inputs to a column consist of afferent fibres from the joint, muscle spindle and skin which are maximally activated by contraction of those muscles innervated by that same area of cortex. So, for example, a group of cortical columns in MsI will receive sensory inputs from a finger when it is flexed — that input being provided by the skin receptors on the front of the finger, the muscle spindles in the finger flexors and the joint receptors of the finger joints. That same column will also send a projection to the motorneurones (MNs) in the spinal cord that innervate the finger flexors. Activation of the corticospinal neurone from that column will ultimately activate the receptors that project to that same column, and vice versa. Thus, each column is said to have **input–output coupling** and this may be important in the more complex reflex control of movement as, for example, with the **long-latency or transcortical reflexes**. These reflexes refer to the delayed and smaller electromyographical (EMG) changes that are seen following the sudden stretch of a muscle — the first EMG change being the M1 response of the monosynaptic stretch reflex (see Chapter 33). The transcortical reflex has as its afferent limb the muscle spindle input via the Ia fibre (relayed via the dorsal column–medial lemniscal pathway) and the efferent pathway involves the corticospinal tract (CoST). The exact role of this reflex is not known but it may be important in controlling movements precisely, especially when unexpected obstacles are encountered which activate the muscle spindle.

There has been great controversy as to whether MsI controls individual muscles, simple movements or some other aspect of movements. Neurones within MsI fire before any EMG changes and appear to **code for the direction and force of a movement**, although this activity is dependent on the nature of the task being performed. Therefore, as a whole, the motor cortex controls movement by its innervation of populations of MNs, as individual corticospinal axons innervate many different MNs.

MsI is capable of being remodelled after lesions or changes in sensory feedback, implying that it maintains a flexible relationship with the muscles throughout life. Thus, cells in a region of MsI can shift from the control of one set of muscles to a new set. Within given areas of cortex there is some evidence that synaptic strengths can be altered with long-term potentiation (see Chapter 45), which suggests that the MsI may be capable of learning new movements, a function traditionally ascribed to the cerebellum (see Chapter 37).

Damage to MsI in isolation is rare and experimentally tends to produce deficiencies similar to those seen with selective pyramidal tract lesions. However, damage to both MsI and adjacent premotor areas, as occurs in most cerebrovascular accidents (CVAs) involving the middle cerebral artery (see Chapter 17), produces a much more significant deficiency, with a significant hemiparesis. In contrast, lesions localized to the SMA produce a distinct picture of bilateral failure to initiate movements, while lesions in the frontal eye field produce restrictions of eye movement.

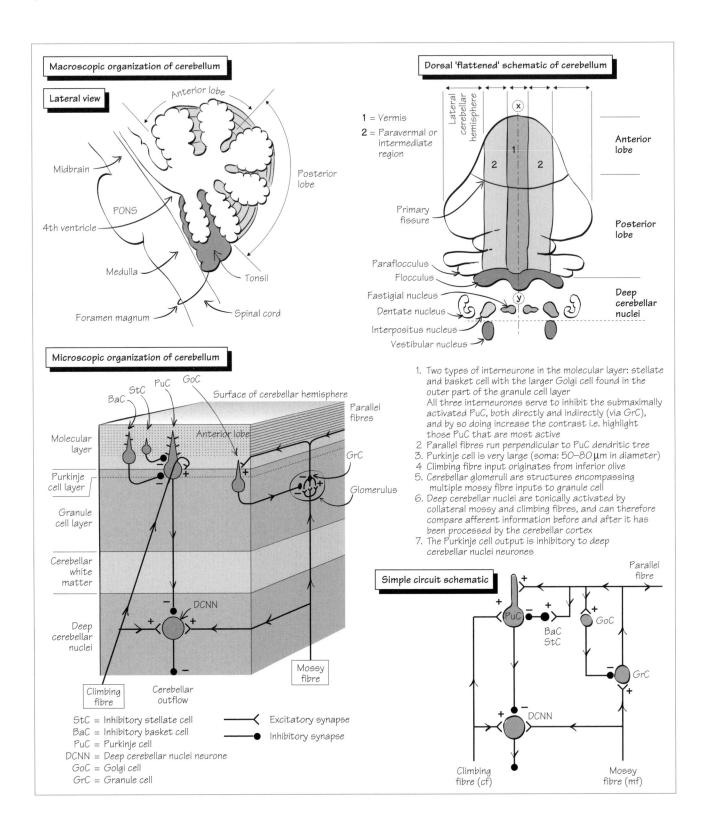

1. Two types of interneurone in the molecular layer: stellate and basket cell with the larger Golgi cell found in the outer part of the granule cell layer
All three interneurones serve to inhibit the submaximally activated PuC, both directly and indirectly (via GrC), and by so doing increase the contrast i.e. highlight those PuC that are most active
2. Parallel fibres run perpendicular to PuC dendritic tree
3. Purkinje cell is very large (soma: 50–80 μm in diameter)
4. Climbing fibre input originates from inferior olive
5. Cerebellar glomeruli are structures encompassing multiple mossy fibre inputs to granule cell
6. Deep cerebellar nuclei are tonically activated by collateral mossy and climbing fibres, and can therefore compare afferent information before and after it has been processed by the cerebellar cortex
7. The Purkinje cell output is inhibitory to deep cerebellar nuclei neurones

Organization of the cerebellum

The **cerebellum (CBM)** is a complex structure found below the tentorial membrane in the posterior fossa and connected to the brainstem by three pairs of (cerebellar) peduncles (see Chapter 13). It is primarily involved in the coordination and learning of movements, and is best thought of in terms of three functional and anatomical systems:

1 spinoCBM—involved with the control of axial musculature and posture ▨ + ▨;

2 pontoCBM—involved with the coordination and planning of limb movements ☐; and

3 vestibuloCBM—involved with posture and the control of eye movements ▪.

These three systems have their own unique pattern of connections (see Appendix 3). The spinoCBM can be divided into a vermal and paravermal (intermediate) region with the former having a close association with the axial musculature. It is therefore associated with the ventromedial descending motor pathways and motorneurones (MNs) while the paravermal part of the spinoCBM is more concerned with the coordination of the limbs. The pontoCBM has a role in this coordination but is more concerned with the visual control of movement by relaying information from the posterior parietal cortex to the motor cortical areas. The vestibuloCBM has no associated deep cerebellar nucleus and is phylogenetically one of the oldest parts of the cerebellum. It, like the vermal part of the spinoCBM, is more concerned with balance through its connections with the ventromedial motor pathways but also has a role in the control of eye movements (see Chapter 40).

In general, the CBM compares the intended movement originating from the motor cortical areas with the actual movement as relayed by the muscle afferents and spinal cord interneurones while receiving an important input from the vestibular and visual system. The comparison having been made, an error signal is relayed via descending motor pathways, and the correction factor stored as part of a motor memory in the synaptic inputs to the Purkinje cell (PuC). This modifiable synapse at the level of the PuC is an example of **long-term depression** (LTD; see Chapters 45 and 47). It describes the reduced synaptic input of the parallel fibre (pf) to PuC when it is activated in phase and at low frequency with the climbing fibre input to that same PuC and which persists for several hours at least. In other words, at times of new movements the climbing fibre input to the PuC increases which has a modifying effect on the pf input to that same PuC. As the movement becomes more routine, the climbing fibre (cf) lessens but the modified (reduced) pf input persists: it is this modification that is thought to underlie the learning and memory of movements.

This modifiable synapse was first proposed by Marr in 1969 and subsequently has been verified, especially with respect to the vestibulo-ocular reflex (see Chapters 28 and 47). The biochemical basis of LTD in the CBM is unknown but appears to rely on the activation of different glutamate receptors in the PuC and the subsequent influx of calcium and the activation of a protein kinase. The presence of a modifiable synapse implies that the CBM is capable of learning and storing information in a motor memory (see Appendix 3).

The microscopic organization of the cerebellum, which allows for the generation of LTD is well characterized, even if the biochemical basis for it remains obscure. The excitatory input to the cerebellum is provided by a mossy and climbing fibre input. The mossy fibre indirectly activates PuC through pfs that originate from granule cells (GrC). In contrast, the climbing fibre directly synapses on the PuC and, as with the mossy fibre input, there is an input to the deep cerebellar nuclei neurones (DCNN). These neurones are therefore tonically excited by the input fibres to the cerebellum, and are inhibited by the output from the cerebellar cortex (the PuC). The PuC in turn are inhibited by a number of local interneurones, while Golgi cells (GoC) in the outer granule cell layer provide an inhibitory input to the GrC. All of these interneurones have the effect of inhibiting submaximally activated PuC and GrC, and by so doing highlight the signal to be analysed.

The final output of the cerebellum from the deep cerebellar nuclei to various brainstem structures is also inhibitory.

Clinical features of cerebellar damage

Much that can be deduced about the function of the CBM is derived from the clinical features of patients with cerebellar damage.

Dysfunction of the CBM is found in a large number of conditions, and the clinical features of cerebellar damage are as follows.

1 Hypotonia or reduced muscle tone. This is caused by a reduced input from the DCNN via the descending motor pathways to the muscle spindle (see Chapter 33).

2 Incoordination/ataxia. There are a number of manifestations of this including: asynergy (an inability to coordinate the contraction of agonist and antagonist muscles); dysmetria (an inability to terminate movements accurately which can result in an intention tremor and past pointing); and dysdiadochokinesis (an inability to perform rapidly alternating movements). Ataxia is often used to describe incoordinated movements. In cases where the vermis is predominantly involved, as occurs in alcoholic cerebellar degeneration, this results in a staggering wide-based 'drunk-like' character to the gait. When there is involvement of the more lateral parts of the cerebellar hemisphere the incoordination involves the limbs.

3 Dysarthria. This is an inability to articulate words properly caused by incoordination of the oropharyngeal musculature. The words are slurred and spoken slowly (scanning dysarthia).

4 Nystagmus. This describes rapid jerky eye movements caused by a breakdown in the outflow from the vestibular nucleus and its connections with the oculomotor nuclei (see Chapters 28 and 40).

5 Palatal tremor or myoclonus. This is a rare condition in which there is hypertrophy of the inferior olive, with damage in a triangle bounded by this structure, the dentate nucleus of the CBM and the red nucleus in the midbrain (Mollaret triangle). The patient characteristically has a low-frequency tremor of the palate, which oscillates up and down.

Finally, there is a recent suggestion that the cerebellum may also subserve some cognitive function as subtle deficits can be seen in this domain in some patients with cerebellar disease.

Function of the cerebellum

The **role of the CBM** can be defined by area and correlates well with the localizing signs of cerebellar disease. Exactly how the CBM achieves these functions is unknown, but the repetition of the same elementary circuitry in all parts of the cerebellar cortex implies a common mode of function. Three possibilities exist which are not mutually exclusive.

1 By acting as a comparator. The CBM compares the descending supraspinal motor signals (efference copy, intended movement) with the ascending afferent feedback information (actual movement), and any discrepancy is corrected by the output of the CBM through descending motor pathways. This allows the CBM to coordinate movements so that they are achieved smoothly and accurately.

2 By acting as a timing device. The CBM (especially the pontoCBM) converts descending motor signals into a sequence of motor activation so that movement is performed in a smooth and coordinated fashion, with balance and posture maintained by the vestibulo- and spinoCBM.

3 By initiating and storing movements. The existence of a modifiable synapse at the level of the PuC means that the CBM is capable of storing motor information and updating it. Therefore, under the appropriate circumstances, the right sequence for a movement can be accessed and fed through the supraspinal motor pathways, and by so doing initiate an accurate learnt movement.

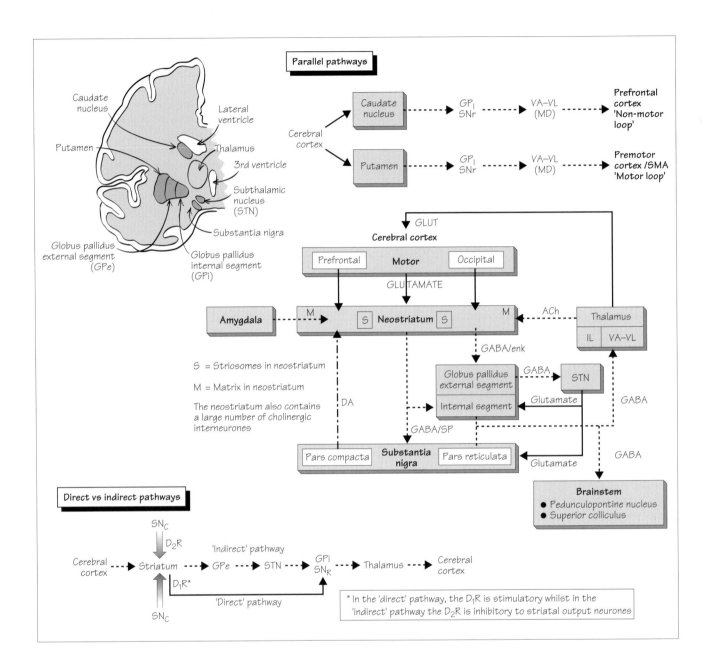

The **basal ganglia** consist of the **caudate and putamen (dorsal or neostriatum; NS)**, the **internal and external segments of the globus pallidus (GPi and GPe**, respectively), the **pars reticulata and pars compacta of the substantia nigra (SNr and SNc**, respectively) and the **subthalamic nucleus (STN)**.

The NS is the main receiving area of the basal ganglia and receives information from the whole cortex in a somatotopic fashion as well as the intralaminar nuclei of the thalamus (IL). The major outflow from the basal ganglia is via the GPi and SNr to the ventroanterior–ventrolateral nuclei of the thalamus (VA–VL) which in turn project to the premotor cortex (PMC), supplementary motor area (SMA) and prefrontal cortex. In addition, there is a projection to the brainstem, especially to the pedunculopontine nucleus (PPN) that is involved in locomotion (see

Chapter 34), and to the superior colliculus that is involved with eye movements (see Chapters 24 and 40).

The basal ganglia also have a **number of loops** within them that are important. There is a striato–nigral–striatal loop with the latter projection being dopaminergic in nature. This pathway degenerates in *Parkinson's disease*. There is also a loop from the GPe to the STN which then projects back to the GPi and SNr. This pathway is excitatory in nature and is important in controlling the level of activation of the inhibitory output nuclei of the basal ganglia to the thalamus. However, although a marked degree of convergence and divergence can be seen throughout the basal ganglia, the projections do form parallel pathways, which at the most simplistic level divide into a motor pathway through the putamen and a non-motor pathway through the caudate nucleus.

The NS consists of **patches or striosomes** that are deficient in the enzyme acetylcholinesterase (AChE). These are embedded in an otherwise AChE-rich striatum, which forms the large extrastriosomal **matrix**. In general, the striosomes are closely related to the dopaminergic nigrostriatal pathway and prefrontal cortex and amygdala, while the matrix is more involved with sensorimotor areas. However, the relationship of these two components of the neostriatum to any parallel pathways is not clear.

This non-motor role of the basal ganglia is perhaps more clearly seen with the **ventral extension of the basal ganglia** which consists of the ventral striatum (nucleus accumbens), ventral pallidum and substantia innominata (not shown in the figure). It receives a dopaminergic input from the ventral tegmental area that lies adjacent to the SNc in the mid-brain. The ventral striatum ultimately projects via the thalamus to the prefrontal cortex and frontal eye fields. These structures are intimately associated with motivation and drug addiction.

The **neurophysiology** of the basal ganglia shows that many of the cells within it have complex properties that are not clearly sensory or motor in terms of their response characteristics. For example, some units in the NS respond to sensory stimuli but only when that sensory stimulus is a trigger for a movement. In contrast, many units in the pallidum respond maximally to movement about a given joint before any electromyographic (EMG) changes. Thus, from a neurophysiological point of view, the basal ganglia take highly processed sensory information and convert it into some form of motor programme. This is supported by the clinical disorders that affect the basal ganglia.

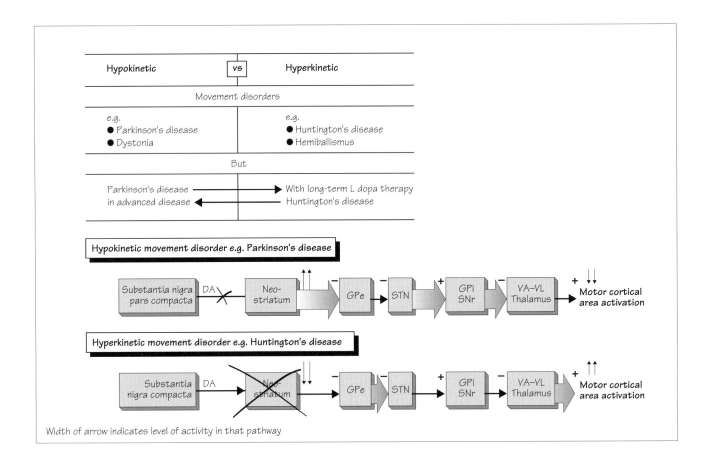

Width of arrow indicates level of activity in that pathway

Parkinson's disease

Parkinson's disease is a degenerative disorder that typically affects people in their sixth and seventh decades of life. The primary pathological event is the loss of the dopaminergic nigrostriatal tract, with the formation of characteristic histological inclusion bodies, known as Lewy bodies. In the vast majority of cases the disease develops for reasons that are not clear (idiopathic Parkinson's disease; see Chapter 52). However, in some cases clear aetiological agents are identified such as vascular lesions in the region of the nigrostriatal pathway, administration of the antidopaminergic drugs in schizophrenia (see Chapter 50) or genetic abnormalities in young patients and some rare families.

Over 50–60% of the dopaminergic nigrostriatal neurones need to be lost before the classical clinical features of idiopathic Parkinson's disease are clearly manifest: slowness to move (bradykinesia); increased tone in the muscles (cogwheel rigidity); and tremor that is present at rest. However, most patients also display a range of cognitive, affective and autonomic abnormalities which may relate to pathological changes at sites other than the nigrostriatal tract.

Neurophysiologically, these patients have increased activity of the neurones in the globus pallidus internal segment (GPi) with a disturbed pattern of discharge, which results from increased activity in the subthalamic nucleus (STN) secondary to the loss of the predominantly inhibitory dopaminergic input to the neostriatum (NS). The increased inhibitory output from the GPi (and presumably the substantia nigra pars reticulata (SNr) as well) to the ventroanterior–ventrolateral nuclei of the thalamus (VA–VL) results in reduced activation of the supplementary motor area (SMA) and other adjacent cortical areas. Thus, patients with Parkinson's disease are unable to initiate movement because of their failure to activate the SMA, although the explanation for the tremor and rigidity is less clear. However, these patients can be treated successfully in the early stages of the disease with various drugs.

Antiparkinsonian drugs

No drug currently has been shown definitely to slow the progression of Parkinson's disease. For most patients, **dopamine replacement therapy** with **levodopa** (L-dopa) or dopamine agonists is the treatment of choice (dopamine itself does not pass the blood–brain barrier). L-dopa is the immediate precursor of dopamine and is converted in the brain by decarboxylation to dopamine. Orally administered L-dopa is largely metabolized outside the brain and so it is given with an extracerebral decarboxylase inhibitor (carbidopa or benserazide), which greatly reduces the effective dose and peripheral adverse effects (e.g. hypotension, nausea). L-dopa frequently produces adverse effects that are mainly caused by widespread stimulation of dopamine receptors. They include nausea and vomiting (as a result of stimulation of the chemoreceptor trigger zone), psychiatric side-effects (e.g. hallucinations, confusion) and dyskinesias. After 5 years' treatment about half the patients will have deteriorated. In some the akinesia gradually recurs, while in others various dyskinesias may appear. The duration of action of each dose of L-dopa may shorten ('end of dose' deterioration) and there may be rapid oscillations in mobility ('on–off' effect).

Selegiline is a selective monoamine oxidase type B (MAO_B) inhibitor that reduces the metabolism of dopamine in the brain and potentiates the action of L-dopa. It may be used in conjunction with L-dopa to reduce 'end of dose' deterioration. **Catecholamine-*O*-methyltransferase (COMT)** inhibitors such as entacapone have recently been developed for use in Parkinson's disease, and they reduce the peripheral metabolism of L-dopa and by so doing increase the amount that can enter the brain.

Dopamine agonists (e.g. ropinirole, cabergoline, pramipexole) are also used often as first-line treatment in young patients or in combination with L-dopa in the later stages of Parkinson's disease in older patients. Dopamine agonists directly bind to the dopamine receptors in the striatum (and substantia nigra) and by so doing activate the postsynaptic output neurones of the striatum. These agents are preferred as the treatment of choice in young-onset Parkinson's disease because of their L-dopa sparing effects which may delay the development of 'on–off' effects.

Other drugs that can be used in Parkinson's disease includes **antimuscarinic drugs** (e.g. trihexyphenidyl (benzhexol), procyclidine) in the early stages where tremor predominates. These drugs are believed to correct a relative overactivity of central cholinergic activation that results from the progressive decrease of (inhibitory) dopaminergic activity. Adverse effects are common and include dry mouth, urinary retention, constipation and confusional states. β-Blockers have also been tried for the tremor of Parkinson's disease with some success.

Although most patients with Parkinson's disease are best treated with drugs, surgical approaches have been undertaken in advanced disease. In Parkinson's disease, there is increased activation of the internal part of the globus pallidus and SNr, which in part is mediated by an input from the excitatory subthalamic nucleus. Recent interest has focused on the surgical manipulation of these basal ganglia nuclei in the form of lesions in the GPi (pallidotomy) or the insertion of electrodes for deep-brain stimulation into the GPi or subthalamic nucleus. This latter approach generates a temporary lesion possibly by inducing a conduction block (see Chapters 6 and 8) and is now probably the surgical treatment of choice in advanced Parkinson's disease. This approach not only seems to ameliorate drug-induced problems but the fundamental motor manifestations of the disease as well. An alternative surgical approach to lesioning or deep-brain stimulation is the implantation of dopamine-rich tissue into the striatum to replace and possibly restore the damaged nigrostriatal pathway. This has been successfully carried out with fetal nigral tissue in a small number of Parkinson's disease patients, although earlier attempts using autografts of the catecholamine-rich adrenal medulla proved unsuccessful. In all cases successful treatment is asso-

ciated with evidence for a reactivation of the appropriate cortical areas but of late there has been concern about side-effects from this treatment including dyskinesias off therapy post-transplantation.

Huntington's disease

Huntington's disease is an inherited autosomal dominant disorder associated with a trinucleotide expansion in the gene coding for the protein huntingtin on chromosome 4 (see Chapter 55).

The disease presents typically in mid life with a progressive dementia and abnormal movements which usually take the form of chorea—rapid dance-like movements, typically of the hands and neck. This type of movement is described as being hyperkinetic in nature, unlike the hypokinetic deficits seen in Parkinson's disease, and reflects the fact that the primary pathology is the loss of the output neurones of the striatum. This results in relative inhibition of the STN and thus reduced inhibitory outflow from the GPi and SNr, which leads to the cortical motor areas being overactivated, generating an excess of movements.

Treatment in Huntington's disease is designed to reduce the level of dopaminergic stimulation within the basal ganglia, but is seldom successful. As in Parkinson's disease, some progress has been made in the possible use of fetal tissue for transplantation into the diseased basal ganglia.

Other disorders of the basal ganglia

Another example of a hyperkinetic movement disorder is *hemiballismus* which is the rapid flailing movements of the limbs contralateral to damage to the subthalamic nucleus.

A number of other conditions can affect the basal ganglia including *Wilson's disease* (an autosomal recessive condition associated with copper deposition); *Sydenham's chorea* (a sequela of rheumatic fever); defects in mitochondrial function (*mitochondrial cytopathies*; see Chapter 55); a number of toxins (e.g. carbon monoxide and manganese) and *choreoathetoid cerebral palsy* (athetosis is defined as an abnormal involuntary slow writhing movement).

The spectrum of movement disorders seen with these diseases is variable because the damage is rarely confined to one structure so patients may exhibit either *parkinsonism, chorea* and *ballismus*, or *dystonia*, where a limb is held in an abnormal fixed posture.

Many of these conditions, including Parkinson's disease and Huntington's disease, have a degree of cognitive impairment—if not frank dementia—and while this may relate to coincidental damage in the cerebral cortex, there is increasing evidence that it may be as a direct result of basal ganglia damage. In this respect the ventral extension of the basal ganglia may be important.

The basal ganglia have a major role in the control of eye movements (see Chapter 40) and so many patients with diseases of the basal ganglia have abnormal eye movements that may be helpful in establishing their clinical diagnosis.

40 Eye movements

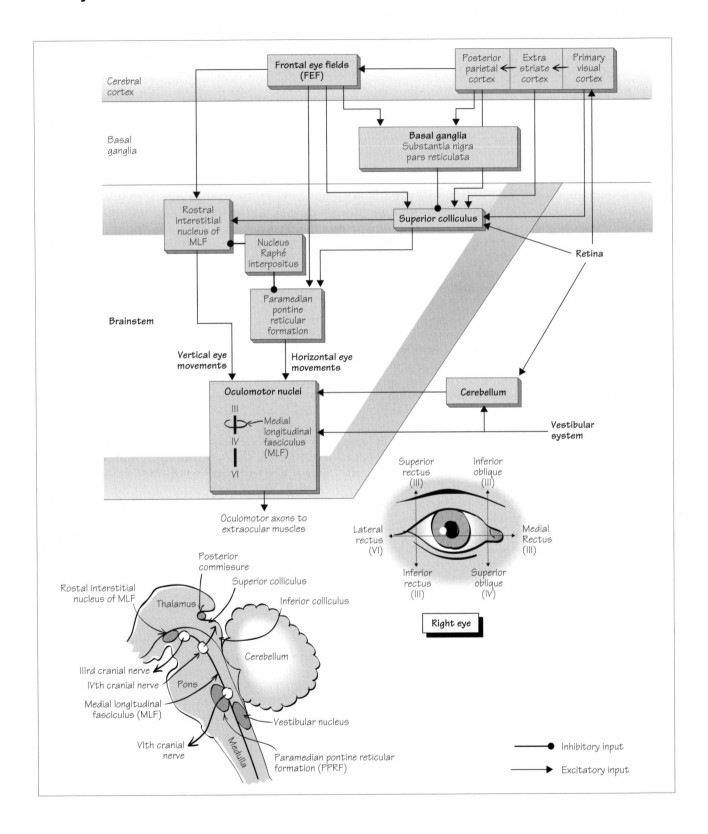

The accurate **control of eye movements** involves a number of different structures, from the extraocular muscles to the frontal cortex and failure to achieve this control results symptomatically in either double vision (diplopia), blurred vision or oscillopsia (perception of an oscillating image or environmental movement). In clinical practice, disruption of the final pathway from the oculomotor nuclei (third, fourth and sixth cranial nerves) to the extraocular muscle represents one of the major causes of diplopia (e.g. *myasthenia gravis*; see Chapter 7), as does inflammation (e.g. *multiple sclerosis*) in the medial longitudinal fasciculus (MLF) pathway linking the oculomotor nuclei.

Types of eye movement

There are three major types of eye movement.

1 Smooth pursuit or the following of a target accurately, which is controlled primarily by posterior parts of the cortex in conjunction with the cerebellum.

2 Saccadic eye movements where there is a sudden shift of the eyes to a new target and which are controlled by more anterior cortical areas, the basal ganglia and superior colliculus in the midbrain.

3 Sustained gaze where the eyes are fixed in one direction and which is primarily a function of the brainstem (especially the paramedian pontine reticular formation (PPRF) and rostral interstitial nucleus of the MLF).

Eye movements, like the motor system in general, can be either **voluntary** (when the command comes from the frontal eye field) or **reflex** (when the command originates from subcortical structures and posterior parietal cortex).

Manifestations of disordered eye movement include a loss of conjugate movements; broken pursuit movements; inaccurate saccades; gaze palsies; and nystagmus. **Nystagmus** is defined as a biphasic ocular oscillation containing an abnormal slow and corrective fast phase, the latter defining the direction of the nystagmus.

Anatomy and physiology of central nervous system control of eye movements

• The **frontal eye fields** (FEF; predominantly Brodmann's area 8) are found anterior to the premotor cortex (PMC; see Chapter 35). Stimulation of this structure produces eye movements, typically saccades, to the contralateral side, and may be seen clinically in some epileptic patients.

Damage to this area reduces the ability to look to the contralateral side so the patient tends to look towards the side of the lesion. The FEF primarily receives from the posterior parietal cortex and projects to the superior colliculus, other brainstem centres and the basal ganglia.

• The **posterior parietal cortex** (corresponds to Brodmann's area 7 in monkeys) contains a large number of neurones responsive to complex visual stimuli, as well as coding for some visually guided eye movements (see Chapter 30). It is especially important in the generation of saccades to objects of visual significance via its connections with the FEF and superior colliculus.

Damage to this area, in addition to causing deficiencies in visual attention and saccades to objects in the contralateral hemifield, can also impair smooth pursuit eye movements as evidenced by loss of the **opto-kinetic reflex**. This is a reflex in which the eyes fixate by a series of rapid movements on a moving target, such as a rotating drum, with vertical lines as fixation targets.

• The **primary visual cortex and its associated extrastriate areas** are involved in both saccadic and smooth pursuit eye movements (see Chapters 24 and 25). The role in saccadic movements is primarily through the projection of V1 to the superior colliculus, while the role in smooth pursuit is via extrastriate area V5 (see Chapter 25), and projections to the FEF, posterior parietal cortex and pons.

Damage to the striate and extrastriate areas, in addition to producing field defects and specific deficiencies of visual function (see Chapter 25), can also cause major abnormalities in smooth pursuit eye movements.

• The **basal ganglia** have a major role in the control of saccadic eye movements (see Chapters 38 and 39). The caudate nucleus receives from the FEF and projects via the substantia nigra pars reticulata to the superior colliculus.

Abnormalities in saccadic eye movements are seen clinically in a number of basal ganglia disorders. For example, in *Parkinson's disease* the saccadic eye movements tend to be slightly inaccurate with undershooting to the target (hypometric saccades).

• The **superior colliculus** in the midbrain is important in the accurate execution of saccades (see Chapter 24).

• The **cerebellum and vestibular nuclei** have important complex inputs into the brainstem oculomotor system and are especially important in the control of pursuit movements, as well as mediating the vestibulo-ocular reflex (see Chapters 28, 37 and 47).

Damage to the cerebellum and vestibular system causes broken pursuit eye movements, inaccurate saccades and nystagmus.

• The **rostral interstitial nucleus of the medial longitudinal fasciculus (riMLF)** is important in the control of vertical saccades and vertical gaze (both up- and downgaze) and receives important inputs from the FEF and superior colliculus while projecting to all the oculomotor nuclei.

Damage to this structure or disruption of its afferent inputs therefore produces deficiencies in both these eye movements, and this can occur in a number of conditions including some neurodegenerative diseases.

• The **PPRF** receives from the FEF, superior colliculus and cerebellum and is responsible for horizontal saccades and gaze. It is thought that this structure may work in conjunction with another pontine nucleus, the **nucleus raphe interpositus**. This latter nucleus contains omnipause neurones, which normally exert tonic inhibition on the burst neurones of the PPRF (and riMLF) mediating the saccadic impulse.

Damage to nucleus raphe interpositus results in random chaotic eye movements or *opsoclonus*. In contrast, damage to the PPRF causes deficiencies in saccadic eye movements as well as ipsilateral gaze paresis.

• The **MLF** mediates conjugate eye movements through interconnections between all the oculomotor nuclei and is commonly affected in some diseases of the CNS, such as *multiple sclerosis* (see Chapter 54).

A lesion in this structure causes an *internuclear ophthalmoplegia*, with nystagmus in the abducting eye and slowed or absent adduction in the other eye.

41 Clinical disorders of the motor system

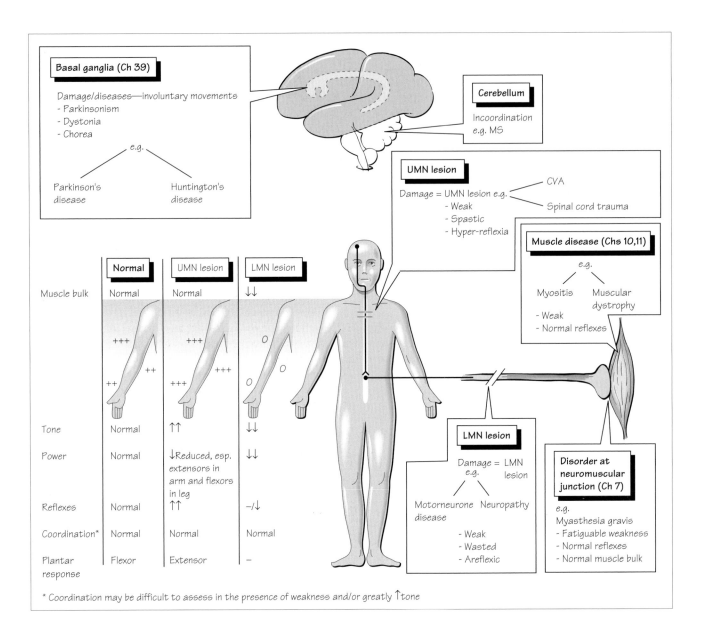

Basal ganglia (Ch 39)

Damage/diseases—involuntary movements
- Parkinsonism
- Dystonia
- Chorea

e.g.

Parkinson's disease   Huntington's disease

Cerebellum

Incoordination
e.g. MS

UMN lesion

Damage = UMN lesion e.g.
- Weak
- Spastic
- Hyper-reflexia

CVA

Spinal cord trauma

Muscle disease (Chs 10,11)

e.g.

Myositis   Muscular dystrophy

- Weak
- Normal reflexes

LMN lesion

Damage = LMN lesion
e.g.

Motorneurone disease   Neuropathy

- Weak
- Wasted
- Areflexic

Disorder at neuromuscular junction (Ch 7)

e.g.
Myasthesia gravis
- Fatiguable weakness
- Normal reflexes
- Normal muscle bulk

	Normal	UMN lesion	LMN lesion
Muscle bulk	Normal	Normal	↓↓
Tone	Normal	↑↑	↓↓
Power	Normal	↓Reduced, esp. extensors in arm and flexors in leg	↓↓
Reflexes	Normal	↑↑	–/↓
Coordination*	Normal	Normal	Normal
Plantar response	Flexor	Extensor	–

* Coordination may be difficult to assess in the presence of weakness and/or greatly ↑tone

Disturbances in the motor pathways can produce a range of disorders of movement. These typically involve the muscle causing weakness; the neuromuscular junction (NMJ) causing fatiguable weakness; the motorneurones (lower or upper) giving weakness and changes in muscle tone and reflexes; the cerebellum and its connections causing problems with coordination without any changes in power or reflexes; and the basal ganglia which produces an abnormal involuntary movement without any effect on power, reflexes or coordination.

In order to determine the nature and cause of the motor disturbance a full history and examination is needed along with appropriate tests. The majority of patients with isolated motor symptoms have either Parkinson's or motorneurone disease, although by far the most common clinical scenario is the patient with both motor and sensory abnormalities as a result of strokes or damaged nerves as they emerge or pass along the limb.

A typical screen of tests for patients with motor symptoms involves blood tests, nerve conduction studies (NCS), electromyography (EMG) and magnetic resonance imaging (MRI) of brain and spinal cord.

Muscle (see Chapters 10 and 11)

The typical features of a muscle disease are weakness, which may relate to exercise, and on occasions muscle pain (myalgia). The age and rate of progression is often helpful in determining the type of muscle disease, e.g. progressive slow weakness without pain from childhood would suggest a degenerative *muscular dystrophy* (see Chapter 10) while a short history of painful weakness in adulthood would suggest an *inflammatory myositis* (see Chapter 54). The distribution of weakness is also helpful in defining the likely type of muscle disease, e.g. proximal arm and leg weakness in *limb girdle muscular dystrophy*. The investigations that are especially useful in muscle disease are muscle-specific creatine phosphokinase (CPK)—a measure of muscle damage; EMG and muscle biopsy. In some cases genetic testing is of value, especially if the muscle weakness is associated with myotonia and the other features of *myotonic dystrophy*.

Neuromuscular junction (see Chapter 7)

Patients with these disorders present with a history of weakness that gets worse with continued use of the muscle. The most common disorder of the NMJ is *myasthenia gravis*, which typically presents in early or late adulthood with fatiguable diplopia, ptosis, facial and bulbar weakness and proximal limb weakness. The examination confirms weakness that may be present at rest but clearly gets worse with exercise. Patients can present as a neurological emergency if there is bulbar and respiratory failure. Diagnosis typically relies on history and examination, the presence of acetylcholine receptor (AChR) or muscle-specific kinase (MUSK) antibodies, a positive response to a short-acting acetylcholinesterase inhibitor (Tensilon test) and abnormalities on repetitive stimulation with NCS and EMG. Muscle biopsy is not necessary. In some patients myasthenia gravis is associated with either enlargement (hyperplasia) or a tumour of the thymus gland. Other myasthenic syndromes are rare.

Peripheral nerve

Damage to the peripheral nerves will generally give both sensory and motor symptoms and signs. However, the peripheral motor nerve can be preferentially involved in some neuropathies as well as in conditions such as *poliomyelitis* and *motorneurone disease*, which target the actual motorneurone cell body in the ventral horn of the spinal cord and/or brainstem. The typical features of damage to the peripheral motor nerve are weakness, wasting, fasciculation and loss of reflexes — a lower motorneurone (LMN) lesion. Investigation of LMN syndromes involves excluding nerve entrapment as it comes out of the spinal cord by MRI imaging, along with NCS and EMG—the latter showing features of denervation with spontaneous motor discharges from the muscle that has lost its normal innervation.

Spinal cord

The involvement of spinal cord pathways gives a variety of motor syndromes (see Chapter 34). In rare cases there is involvement of spinal cord interneurones giving continuous motor unit activity (CMUA) and a *stiff-man syndrome* (see Chapter 34). Involvement of descending motor pathways from the brain in the spinal cord gives an upper motorneurone (UMN) syndrome of weakness, spasticity, increased reflexes, and clonus and extensor plantars. It is unusual for this pathway to be selectively involved in spinal cord pathology and when it is the patient often also has LMN signs and has a form of motorneurone disease called *amyotrophic lateral sclerosis or Lou Gehrig disease*. Structural lesions of the spinal cord typically produce a combination of motor and sensory signs and symptoms. Investigation involves MRI, with cerebrospinal fluid (CSF) examination if an inflammatory aetiology is suspected and in some cases neurophysiological testing with EMG, NCS and central motor conduction time (CMCT).

Brain

Damage to supraspinal structures can produce a variety of motor signs and symptoms. Involvement is most commonly seen in *cerebrovascular accidents (CVAs)* with involvement of all the descending motor pathways from the cortex to the brainstem and spinal cord. This gives rise to a contralateral hemiparesis with UMN signs. If the left hemisphere is involved there is typically a major disturbance in speech. Occasionally, damage is restricted to the motor cortex, when the patient may present with focal motor seizures such as *Jacksonian epilepsy* (see Chapters 35 and 36). The mainstay of investigation of supraspinal motor abnormalities is MRI/computerized tomography (CT) imaging and CSF examination if an inflammatory aetiology is suspected. In some cases genetic testing is helpful.

Other sites commonly involved in disease processes
Basal ganglia

Produces either a slowness of movement such as in *Parkinson's disease*; an abnormality of limb posture and movement (*dystonia*) or the development of uncontrollable involuntary movements such as *chorea* and *hemiballismus* (see Chapter 39).

Cerebellum

Produces incoordination of movement with slurred speech and abnormal eye movements (see Chapter 37). The disease processes that typically affect this part of the CNS are *multiple sclerosis*, drugs such as anticonvulsants, and alcohol. It can also be involved by tumour growth in which case the situation may be complicated by the development of *hydrocephalus* through compression of the fourth ventricle and its outflow foramina (see Chapter 16).

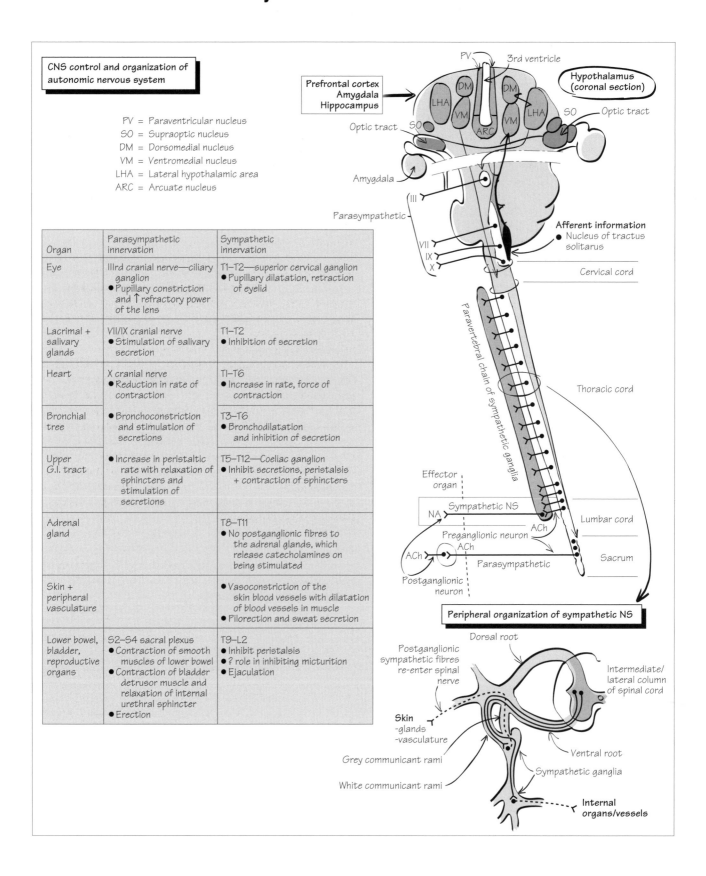

CNS control and organization of autonomic nervous system

PV = Paraventricular nucleus
SO = Supraoptic nucleus
DM = Dorsomedial nucleus
VM = Ventromedial nucleus
LHA = Lateral hypothalamic area
ARC = Arcuate nucleus

Organ	Parasympathetic innervation	Sympathetic innervation
Eye	IIIrd cranial nerve—ciliary ganglion • Pupillary constriction and ↑refractory power of the lens	T1–T2—superior cervical ganglion • Pupillary dilatation, retraction of eyelid
Lacrimal + salivary glands	VII/IX cranial nerve • Stimulation of salivary secretion	T1–T2 • Inhibition of secretion
Heart	X cranial nerve • Reduction in rate of contraction	T1–T6 • Increase in rate, force of contraction
Bronchial tree	• Bronchoconstriction and stimulation of secretions	T3–T6 • Bronchodilatation and inhibition of secretion
Upper G.I. tract	• Increase in peristaltic rate with relaxation of sphincters and stimulation of secretions	T5–T12—Coeliac ganglion • Inhibit secretions, peristalsis + contraction of sphincters
Adrenal gland		T8–T11 • No postganglionic fibres to the adrenal glands, which release catecholamines on being stimulated
Skin + peripheral vasculature		• Vasoconstriction of the skin blood vessels with dilatation of blood vessels in muscle • Pilorection and sweat secretion
Lower bowel, bladder, reproductive organs	S2–S4 sacral plexus • Contraction of smooth muscles of lower bowel • Contraction of bladder detrusor muscle and relaxation of internal urethral sphincter • Erection	T9–L2 • Inhibit peristalsis • ? role in inhibiting micturition • Ejaculation

Prefrontal cortex
Amygdala
Hippocampus

PV
3rd ventricle
DM
DM
LHA
LHA
Hypothalamus (coronal section)
VM
VM
SO
Optic tract
ARC
Optic tract
SO

Amygdala

III

Parasympathetic

VII
IX
X

Afferent information
• Nucleus of tractus solitarus

Cervical cord

Paravertebral chain of sympathetic ganglia

Thoracic cord

Effector organ

NA
Sympathetic NS

Lumbar cord

Preganglionic neuron
ACh

ACh
ACh
Parasympathetic

Sacrum

Postganglionic neuron

Peripheral organization of sympathetic NS

Dorsal root

Postganglionic sympathetic fibres re-enter spinal nerve

Intermediate/lateral column of spinal cord

Skin
-glands
-vasculature

Grey communicant rami

Ventral root

Sympathetic ganglia

White communicant rami

Internal organs/vessels

Anatomy of the autonomic nervous system

The **autonomic nervous system (ANS)** includes those nerve cells and fibres that innervate internal and glandular organs. They subserve the regulation of processes that usually are not under voluntary influence. The **efferent conducting pathway** from the central nervous system (CNS) to the innervated organ always consists of two succeeding neurones: one **preganglionic** and the other **postganglionic**, with the former having its cell body in the CNS (see Chapter 1).

The ANS is subdivided into the **enteric**, **sympathetic** and **parasympathetic nervous systems** with the latter two systems commonly exerting opposing influences on the structure they are both innervating. The sympathetic nervous system preganglionic neurones are found in the intermediate part (lateral horn) of the spinal cord from the upper thoracic to mid-lumbar cord (T1–L3). The preganglionic parasympathetic neurones have their cell bodies in the brainstem and sacrum. The postganglionic cell bodies are found in the vertebral and prevertebral ganglia in the sympathetic nervous system but in the parasympathetic system they are situated either adjacent to or in the walls of the organ they supply.

In addition to these anatomical differences there are pharmacological ones, with the sympathetic nervous system using **noradrenaline** (norepinephrine; NA) as its postganglionic transmitter while the parasympathetic nervous system uses **acetylcholine** (ACh). Both systems use ACh at the level of the ganglia.

Central nervous system control of the autonomic nervous system

The **CNS control of the ANS** is complex, involving a number of brainstem structures as well as the **hypothalamus** (see Chapter 43). The main hypothalamic areas involved in the control of the ANS are the ventromedial hypothalamic area in the case of the sympathetic nervous system and the lateral hypothalamic area in the parasympathetic nervous system. These controlling pathways can be direct or indirect via a number of brainstem structures such as the periaqueductal grey matter and parts of the reticular formation (see Chapter 13).

Clinical features of damage to the autonomic nervous system

Damage to the ANS can either be local to a given anatomical structure, or generalized when there is loss of the whole system caused by either a central or peripheral disease process. **Focal** peripheral lesions are not uncommon and the deficiencies resulting from these lesions can be easily predicted. For example, loss of the sympathetic innervation to the eye results in pupillary constriction (miosis), drooping of the upper eyelid (ptosis) and loss of sweating around the eye (anhydrosis)—a triad of signs known as *Horner's syndrome*. Other examples include the *reflex sympathetic dystrophies* where there is severe pain and autonomic changes confined to a single limb, often in response to some trivial injury (see Chapter 22). The exact role of the sympathetic nervous system in the genesis of these conditions is not known, as local sympathectomies are not always effective treatment and this condition has now been renamed complex regional pain syndrome. However, in some instances the nociceptors start expressing receptors for noradrenaline (norepinephrine) (see Chapter 22).

More **global** damage to the ANS can occur because of degeneration of the central neurones either in isolation (e.g. *pure autonomic failure*) or as part of a more widespread degenerative process as is seen, e.g. in *multiple-system atrophy* where there may be additional cell loss in the basal ganglia and cerebellum. Alternatively, the autonomic failure may result from a loss of the peripheral neurones, e.g. in diabetes mellitus, alcoholism and *Guillain–Barré syndrome*.

In all these cases the patient presents with orthostatic and postprandial hypotension (syncopal or presyncopal symptoms on standing, exercising or eating a big meal) with a loss of variation in heart rate, bowel and bladder disturbances (urinary urgency, frequency and incontinence), impotence and loss of sweating and pupillary responses. The symptoms are often difficult to treat and a number of agents are employed to try to improve the postural hypotension and sphincter abnormalities. Such agents for postural hypotension include fludrocortisone, ephedrine, midodrine and vasopressin analogues (all of which cause fluid retention) and cisapride (a potentiator of ACh release) for the gastrointestinal paresis.

43 The hypothalamus

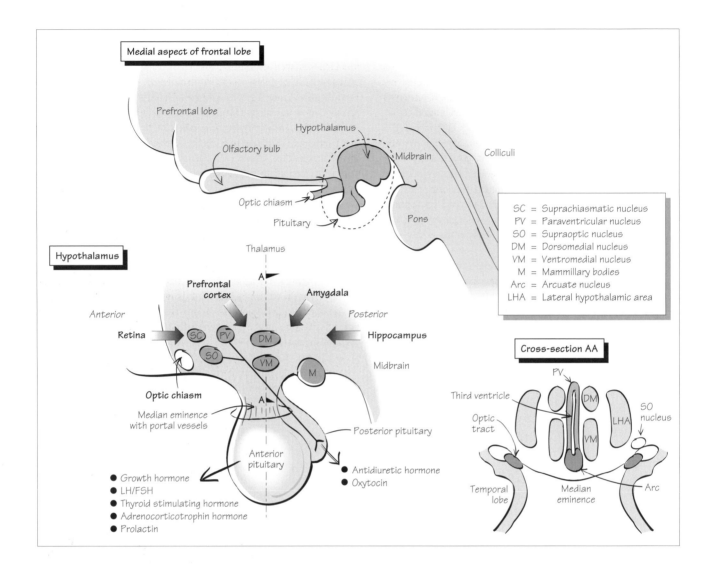

Medial aspect of frontal lobe

Prefrontal lobe
Hypothalamus
Olfactory bulb
Midbrain
Colliculi
Optic chiasm
Pituitary
Pons

SC = Suprachiasmatic nucleus
PV = Paraventricular nucleus
SO = Supraoptic nucleus
DM = Dorsomedial nucleus
VM = Ventromedial nucleus
M = Mammillary bodies
Arc = Arcuate nucleus
LHA = Lateral hypothalamic area

Hypothalamus

Thalamus
Prefrontal cortex
Amygdala
Anterior
Posterior
Retina
Hippocampus
Midbrain
Optic chiasm
Median eminence with portal vessels
Posterior pituitary
Anterior pituitary
● Growth hormone
● LH/FSH
● Thyroid stimulating hormone
● Adrenocorticotrophin hormone
● Prolactin
● Antidiuretic hormone
● Oxytocin

Cross-section AA

Third ventricle
PV
DM
Optic tract
SO nucleus
LHA
VM
Temporal lobe
Median eminence
Arc

The hypothalamus lies on either side of the third ventricle, below the thalamus and between the optic chiasm and the midbrain, and receives a significant input from limbic system structures (see Chapter 45). It also receives from the retina, as well as containing a large number of neurones that are sensitive to changes in hormone levels, electrolyte changes and temperature changes. In addition to an efferent output to the autonomic nervous system (ANS), it has a critical role in the control of pituitary endocrine function (a detailed discussion on the endocrinology of the hypothalamic–pituitary system is beyond the scope of this book).

Thus, the hypothalamus, while being important in the control of the ANS, has a much greater role in the homoeostasis of many physiological systems (e.g. thirst, hunger, sodium and water balance, temperature regulation), the control of circadian and endocrine functions, the ability to form anterograde memories (in conjunction with the limbic system; see Chapter 45) and the translation of the response to emotional stimuli into endocrinological and autonomic responses.

The hypothalamus performs a number of other functions, all of which can be lost or deranged in the disease state. The most common cause is as a side-effect of surgical removal of *pituitary tumours*.

The **functions of the hypothalamus** are as follows.

1 It controls the ANS and damage to it can cause autonomic instability. The ventromedial part of the hypothalamus has a major role in controlling the sympathetic nervous system while the lateral hypothalamic area controls the parasympathetic nervous system (see Chapter 42).

2 It controls the endocrine functions of the pituitary by the production of releasing and inhibiting hormones as well as producing antidiuretic hormone (ADH, also known as vasopressin) and oxytocin. Hypothalamic damage can have profound systemic effects because of the endocrinological disturbances associated with it, of which perhaps the most common example is **diabetes insipidus** where there is loss of ADH. In this condition the patient passes many litres of urine each day, which needs to be compensated for by increased fluid intake.

3 The hypothalamus has a major role in coordinating autonomic and

endocrinological responses, both under physiologically appropriate conditions, as well as in the expression of emotional states as coded for by the limbic system. In cases of hypovolaemia or extreme anxiety, for example, the hypothalamus not only mediates increased sympathetic activity but also enhanced cortisol production via the stimulated release of adrenocorticotrophic hormone (ACTH) from the anterior pituitary.

4 It has an important role in thermoregulation. Lesions to the anterior hypothalamic area cause hyperthermia, while stimulation of this same area lowers body temperature via the ANS, in contrast to the posterior hypothalamic area, which behaves in an opposite fashion. It may also mediate some of the more long-term changes seen with prolonged changes in ambient temperature, such as increased thyrotrophin-releasing hormone (TRH) production in patients exposed to a chronically cold enviroment. Damage to the hypothalamus can lead to profound changes in the central control of temperature. In septic states the production of some cytokines (e.g. interleukin-1) may reset the thermostat in the hypothalamus to a higher than normal temperature, accounting for the paradoxical situation of a fever with physiological evidence of mechanisms designed to conserve or generate heat (e.g. shivering).

5 It has a role in the control of feeding. In simple terms, the ventromedial hypothalamus is often called the satiety centre, in that damage to it causes excessive eating (hyperphagia) and weight gain, while damage to the lateral hypothalamic (or hunger) area produces aphagia (no eating at all). The control of these centres involves a number of hormones, including insulin and the more recently described leptins.

6 It has a role in the control of thirst and water balance by virtue of its osmoreceptors; the afferent input from a host of peripheral sensory receptors (e.g. atrial stretch receptors in the heart, arterial baroreceptors); the activation of hypothalamic hormone receptors (e.g. angiotensin II receptors); and its efferent output via the ANS to the heart and kidney as well as the production of ADH.

7 It has a role in the control of circadian rhythms via the retinal input to the suprachiasmatic nucleus. This nucleus appears to be critical in setting the circadian rhythm as lesion and transplant experiments have shown. Although the exact mechanism by which these rhythms are mediated is not known, it may involve the production of melatonin by the pineal gland.

8 It has a role with the limbic system in memory. Damage to the mammillary bodies, which receive a significant input from the hippocampal complex as occurs in chronic alcoholism with thiamine deficiency, produces a profound amnesia *(**Korsakoff's syndrome**)* of both an anterograde (inability to lay down new memories) and retrograde (inability to recover old memories) nature. The latter feature distinguishes these patients from those who have hippocampal damage (see Chapter 45) and may explain why patients with Korsakoff's syndrome tend to invent missing information (confabulation).

9 The hypothalamus may also have a role in sexual and emotional behaviour independent of its endocrinological influences.

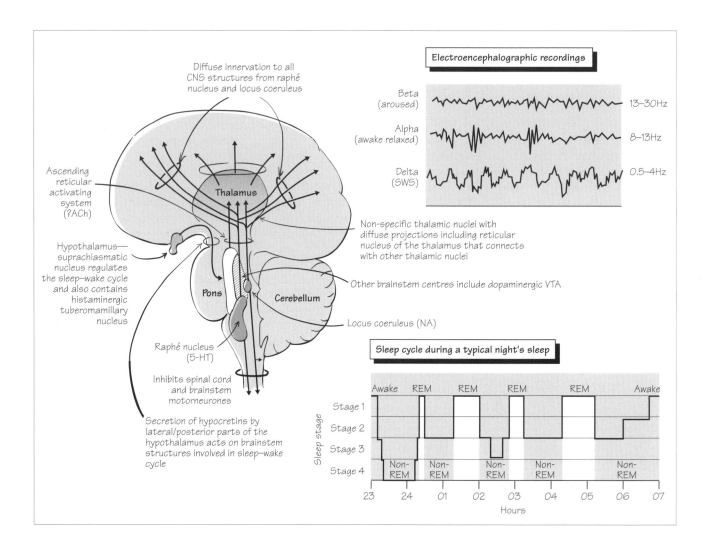

Sleep

Sleep is a characteristic of all mammals and is defined behaviourally as a reduced responsiveness to environmental stimuli, and electrophysiologically by specific changes in electroencephalographic (EEG) activity. In addition, there are a number of changes associated with autonomic nervous system (ANS) function.

Normal patterns of sleep are essential for human well-being, although it is still unclear why we need to dream.

EEG patterns during states of consciousness and slow-wave sleep

EEG recordings from normal awake subjects at rest show a characteristic high-frequency (13–30 Hz, β activity) low-voltage pattern. This desynchronized activity changes as the subject closes his or her eyes and becomes drowsy, with the new EEG pattern having a lower frequency (8–13 Hz, α activity) but slightly higher voltage. This pattern is said to be synchronized and results from the simultaneous firing of many cortical neurones following thalamocortical activity.

EEG studies have revealed that sleep occurs in characteristic stages. As the subject falls asleep (stage 1) the EEG is similar to the awake EEG (low-voltage, fast activity). As sleep deepens through stages 2 and 3 to stage 4, the EEG amplitude progressively increases and its frequency falls. Stage 3 and 4 sleep is called collectively slow-wave sleep (SWS) or **non-rapid eye movement** (non-REM) sleep because the eyes are still. After about 90 min of sleep, the EEG changes back to a low-voltage, fast pattern that is indistinguishable from stage 1 non-REM sleep. However, during this phase of sleep there are rapid eye movements. This type of sleep is called **rapid eye movement sleep** (REM sleep), or paradoxical sleep because although the EEG is similar to that of an awake person, sleepers are difficult to arouse and muscle tone is absent. It is during REM sleep that most dreaming occurs.

Neural mechanisms of sleep

Sleep is an active process, and cholinergic neurones in the brainstem (forming part of the **ascending reticular activating system**) have been shown not only to regulate the desynchronized EEG of the awake state and REM sleep but also to produce pontine–geniculo-occipital (PGO) waves signalling the onset of REM sleep. In contrast, serotonin (5-hydroxytryptamine; 5-HT) containing neurones in the **raphe nuclei** appear to suppress this activity, suggesting that two pharmacologically different systems are responsible for initiating and terminating REM sleep. In addition, noradrenaline-containing neurones in the **locus ceruleus** are responsible for reducing spinal motorneurone excitability producing the associated atonia observed during REM sleep, while the preoptic area and the suprachiasmatic nuclei of the **hypothalamus** are involved in controlling the sleep–wake cycle. Other brainstem and hypothalmic systems are also thought to be important, including the dopaminergic ventral tegmental area and histaminergic tuberomammillary nucleus.

Sleep disorders

Insomnia is the most common sleep disorder. It can be defined as the failure to obtain the required amount or quality of sleep to function normally during the day. ***Primary insomnia*** supposedly brought about by dysfunction of sleep mechanisms in the brain is rare, but these patients are the ones who may require treatment with hypnotic drugs. Causes of secondary insomnia include psychiatric disease (especially depression and anxiety disorders), physical disorders, chronic pain, drug misuse (e.g. excessive alcohol, caffeine), personal crises and old age.

Sleep peptides

More recently a number of peptides have been identified as being associated with sleep states (e.g. delta sleep inducing peptide DSIP). It is unclear what relationship these peptides have with the neural mechanisms described above.

Management of insomnia

Hypnotics are drugs that promote sleep. They include benzodiazepines, chloral hydrate, chlormethiazole and barbiturates. **Benzodiazepines** are by far the most widely used hypnotics. They also have anxiolytic, anticonvulsant, muscle relaxant and amnesic actions. All the actions of benzodiazepines are believed to be caused by the enhancement of γ-aminobutyric acid (GABA) mediated inhibition in the central nervous system (CNS). $GABA_A$ receptors possess several 'modulatory' sites including one for benzodiazepines, which when activated causes a conformational change in the GABA receptor. This increases the affinity of GABA binding and enhances the actions of GABA on the Cl^- conductance of the neuronal membrane.

Any benzodiazepine given at night will induce sleep but a rapidly eliminated drug (e.g. **temazepam**) is usually preferred to avoid daytime sedation. Some newer drugs do not have the benzodiazepine structure but are benzodiazepine-receptor agonists, e.g. **zopiclone** is a cyclopyrrolone with a short duration of action. The benzodiazepines are central depressants but their maximum effect when given orally does not nor-mally cause fatal respiratory depression (in contrast to opioids or barbiturates). Adverse effects include drowsiness, impaired alertness and ataxia as well as a low-grade dependence after a few weeks' use. Withdrawal of the drug may cause a physical withdrawal syndrome (anxiety, insomnia) which may last for weeks.

For many cases of insomnia, psychological strategies may be effective alternatives to drugs.

Hypersomnia (daytime sleepiness)

This is a serious but less common complaint than insomnia. Common causes of persistent daytime sleepiness include narcolepsy, obstructive sleep apnoea, drugs (e.g. benzodiazepines, alcohol, etc.) and depression (20% have hypersomnia rather than insomnia).

Narcolepsy

Narcolepsy is characterized by irresistable sleep episodes lasting 5–30 min during the day and cataplexy (loss of muscle tone and temporary paralysis) usually provoked by emotion, e.g. laughter, anger as well as sleep paralysis and hallucinations at the time of going to or waking up from sleep. It has a very strong HLA association (DR2/DQW1) and, while no pathological abnormalities have been detected in these patients, it is probable that there are abnormalities in the brainstem structures underlying sleep, as there is evidence of short latency REM sleep during normal waking hours. In addition, the identification of the novel neuropeptides **hypocretins or orexins** may be important, as these substances are synthesized in the hypothalamus and act on a number of brainstem centres important in the regulation of sleep. Furthermore, deficiencies in these peptides have recently been described in narcolepsy in some patients and a number of animal models. The syndrome has a devastating effect on quality of life, which may be improved by long-term treatment with stimulants, e.g. dexamfetamine, methylphenidate and modafinil. Clomipramine is used to treat the cataplexy.

Obstructive sleep apnoea syndrome

This occurs if the upper airway at the back of the throat collapses when the patient breathes during sleep. This reduces the oxygen in the blood, which arouses the patient causing him or her to momentarily awake and prevents a normal sleep pattern. The patient, usually an overweight man, is often unaware of these awakenings, but the disruption to sleep results in daytime sleepiness and impaired daytime performance. It can be treated by weight loss, positive ventilatory support at night and, occasionally, oropharyngeal surgery.

45 The limbic system, long-term potentiation and memory

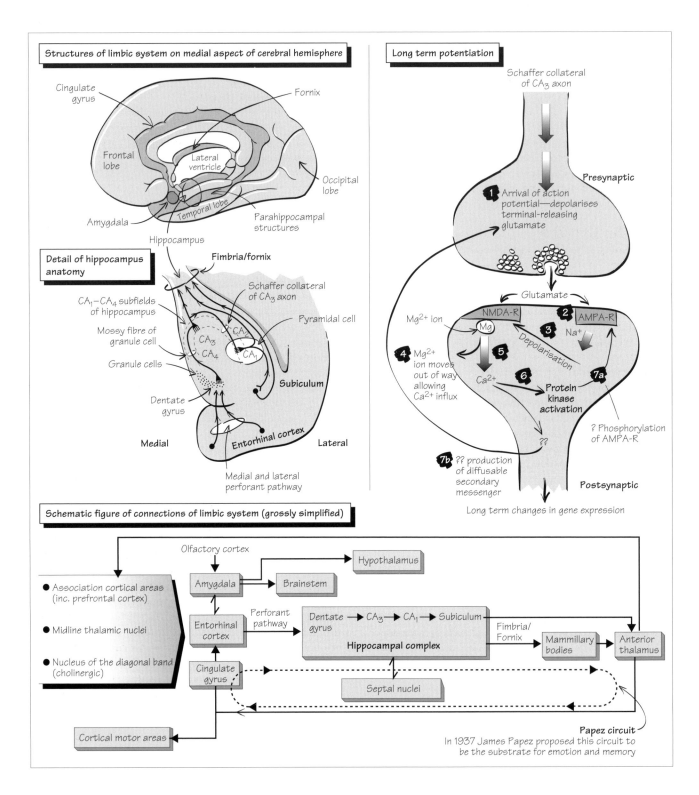

Anatomy of the limbic system

The **limbic system** refers to a collection of areas that lie primarily along the medial aspect of the temporal lobe and includes the **cingulate gyrus**, **parahippocampal structures** (postsubiculum, parasubiculum, presubiculum and perirhinal cortex), **entorhinal cortex**, **hippocampal complex** (dentate gyrus, CA1–CA4 subfields and subiculum), **septal nuclei** and **amygdala**. Additional structures closely associated with it include the mammillary bodies of the hypothalamus, olfactory cortex and nucleus accumbens (see Chapters 43, 29 and 38, respectively).

The **anatomical organization** of the limbic system indicates that it performs some high-level processing of sensory information, given its input from the association cortices (see Chapter 30). The predominant outflow of the limbic system is to the prefrontal cortex and hypothalamus as well as to cortical areas involved with the planning of behaviour, including motor response (see Chapters 32 and 35). Thus, anatomically the limbic system appears to have a role in attaching a behavioural significance and response to a stimulus, especially with respect to its emotional content, and consequently damage to it has profound effects on the emotional responsiveness of the animal. The hippocampal complex has been shown to have both a high degree of susceptibility to hypoxia and yet a remarkable degree of plasticity which helps explain why this structure is important in the generation of epileptic seizures (see Chapter 53) as well as memory acquisition. It is also one of the major sites for neurogenesis in the adult brain, which may also be important in this mnemonic function.

Function of the limbic system

Hippocampal complex and parahippocampal structures

The original description in the 1950s by Scoville and Milner of patient H.M. with bilateral anterior temporal lobectomy for intractable epilepsy and a resulting profound amnesic state suggested that this area of the brain had a major role in memory. Subsequently, the hippocampus proper and parahippocampal areas have been shown to be critical in the ability of both experimental animals and patients to acquire information about events (declarative memory).

However, the long-term storage of memories occurs at a site distant and is probably within the overlying cerebral cortex—as demonstrated by the pattern of memory loss seen in *dementia of the Alzheimer type* (DAT; see Chapter 52). In this condition there is relatively well-preserved retrograde memory (for distant events such as childhood) in the face of severely impaired or absent anterograde memory (inability to remember what the patient has just done).

Amygdala

The amygdala is a small almond-shaped structure made up of many nuclei, that lies on the medial aspect of the temporal lobe and which is involved in the learning and possible storage of emotional aspects of experience.

Damage to this structure experimentally leads to blunted emotional reactions to normally arousing stimuli, and can even prevent the acquisition of emotional behaviour. In humans with selective amygdala damage there appears to be a profound impairment in the ability to recognize facial expressions of fear. Conversely, stimulation of this structure produces a pattern of behaviour typical of fear with increased autonomic activity. This is sometimes seen clinically in *temporal lobe epilepsy* where patients complain of brief episodes of fear.

Cingulate gyrus

The cingulate gyrus running around the medial aspect of the whole hemisphere has a number of functions, including a role in complex motor control (see Chapter 35), pain perception (see Chapters 21 and 22) and social interactions.

Damage to this structure can produce motor neglect, as well as reduced pain perception, reduced aggressiveness and vocalization, emotional blunting and altered social behaviour which can result in a clinical state of *akinetic mutism* (not talking or moving). Stimulation of this area, either experimentally or during an epileptic seizure, produces alterations in the autonomic outflow and motor arrest, with vocalization and complex movements.

Long-term potentiation

Long-term potentiation (LTP) is defined as an increase in the strength of synaptic transmission with repetitive use that lasts for more than a few minutes, and in the hippocampus it can be triggered by less than 1 s of intense synaptic activity and lasts for hours or much longer. It can be induced at a number of central nervous system (CNS) sites but especially the hippocampus and it has therefore been postulated to be important in **memory acquisition**. However, it should be realized that different mechanisms may underlie LTP at different synapses within the hippocampal complex, and that most of the work is based on the excitatory glutamate synapse containing the *N*-methyl-D-aspartate (NMDA) glutamate receptor (NMDA-R; see Chapter 9) in the CA1 subfield of the hippocampal complex.

The current model of LTP is as follows.
- An afferent burst of activity leads to the release of glutamate from the presynaptic terminal (stage 1 on figure).
- The released glutamate then binds to both NMDA and non-NMDA receptors in the postsynaptic membrane. These latter receptors lead to a Na^+ influx (stage 2) which depolarizes the postsynaptic membrane (stage 3).
- The depolarization of the postsynaptic membrane leads not only to an excitatory postsynaptic potential (EPSP), but also removes Mg^{2+} from the NMDA-associated ion channel (stage 4). The Mg^{2+} normally blocks the NMDA receptor associated ion channel and thus its removal in response to postsynaptic depolarization allows a further Na^+ and Ca^{2+} influx into the postsynaptic cell (stage 5).
- The Ca^{2+} influx leads to the activation of a postsynaptic protein kinase (stage 6), which is responsible for the initial **induction of LTP**—a postsynaptic event.
- The **maintenance of LTP**, in addition to requiring a persistent activation of protein kinase activity (stage 7a) the insertion possibly of more postsynaptic glutamate receptors and changes in gene transcription (stage 7c), may also require a modification of neurotransmitter release (stage 7b), i.e. an increase in transmitter release in response to a given afferent impulse. The presynaptic modification, if necessary in the maintenance of LTP, means that the postsynaptic cell must produce a diffusible secondary signal that can act on the presynaptic terminal. Much controversy exists as to the nature of this diffusible messenger, but various candidates have been proposed including permeant arachidonic acid metabolites, nitric oxide, carbon monoxide and platelet activating factor. To date there is no agreement as to which, if any, of these are important in LTP.

In some circumstances **long-term depression (LTD)** can be induced in the mossy fibre synapses in the CA3 subfield of the hippocampus. This, in contrast to LTP, is thought to be mediated by a presynaptic metabotropic glutamate receptor.

46 Neural plasticity and neurotrophic factors I: The peripheral nervous system

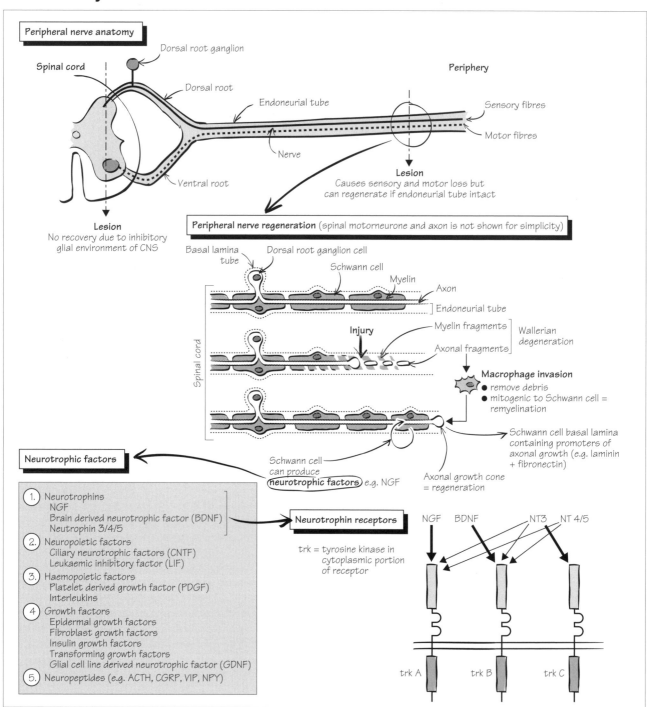

The peripheral nervous system (PNS) is capable of significant repair, to some extent independent of the age at which damage occurs. In contrast, the central nervous system (CNS) has always been thought of as being unable to repair itself although there is now mounting evidence that there is considerable plasticity within it even in the adult state and that most if not all areas of the CNS are capable of some degree of reorganization (see Chapter 47).

Repair in the peripheral nervous system

Injury to a peripheral nerve if severe enough will cause permanent damage with loss of sensation, loss of muscle bulk and weakness. However, in many cases the nerve is able to repair itself, as the peripheral axon can regrow under the influence of the favourable environment of the Schwann cells. This is in contrast to the CNS where the neuroglial cells (astrocytes and oligodendrocytes) are generally inhibitory to axonal growth, even though most CNS neurones are capable of growing new axons.

When a peripheral nerve is damaged, the distal aspect of the axon is lost by a process of **Wallerian degeneration**. Wallerian degeneration leads to the removal and recycling of both axonal and myelin-derived material, but leaves in place dividing Schwann cells inside the basal lamina tube that surrounds all nerve fibres. These columns of Schwann cells surrounded by basal lamina are known as **endoneurial tubes**, and provide the favourable substrate for axonal growth.

Following injury, the degenerating nerve fibre elicits an initial macrophage invasion and this in turn provides the mitogenic input to the Schwann cell. The regenerating axon starts to sprout within hours of injury and contacts the Schwann cell basal laminae on one side, and the Schwann cell membrane on the other. The Schwann cell basal lamina is especially important in the process of axonal sprouting as it contains a number of molecules that are powerful promoters of axonal outgrowth *in vitro* (e.g. laminin and fibronectin).

In addition to providing a favourable substrate for axonal growth, Schwann cells also produce a number of neurotrophic factors, including nerve growth factor (NGF; see below). Thus, the Schwann cell provides a substrate along which the regenerating axon can grow, as well as providing a favourable humoral neurotrophic environment. It also helps direct the regenerating axon back to its appropriate target, by means of the endoneurial tube. Occasionally, the regrowth of the axons is inaccurate or incomplete so, for example, following damage to the third cranial nerve one can have aberrant regeneration such that there is elevation of the eyelid on looking down.

In contrast to axonal damage, the loss of the cell body (in the ventral horn or dorsal root ganglia) leads to an irreversible and permanent loss of axons in the peripheral nerve. Examples of such disorders include *poliomyelitis* and *motorneurone disease (MND)* with respect to the α-MN, and a number of inflammatory and *paraneoplastic syndromes* in the case of the dorsal root ganglia (see Chapters 52 and 54). In all these cases the loss of axons is secondary to the loss of the cell body and so no regeneration is possible. Attempts to rescue dying α-MN in *MND* via the peripheral delivery of neurotrophic factors has been tried without much success (see Chapter 52).

Neurotrophic factors

The number of identified neurotrophic factors has expanded greatly since the original description of the first of these, NGF. These factors, many of which are also found to influence non-neural populations of cells, form discrete families that act through specific types of receptors. Many of these receptors are composed of subunits, one or some of which form common binding domains for a family of neurotrophic factors. For example, the neurotrophin family of neurotrophic factors and the *trk* receptors use a range of cytoplasmic tyrosine kinases as part of their signalling mechanism.

Many populations of neurones respond to neurotrophic factors experimentally both *in vitro* and in the lesioned animal. However, despite these encouraging results, the administration of neurotrophic factors to patients in clinical trials of neurodegenerative disorders and neuropathies has met with only limited success. This argues against these disorders being the result of specific neurotrophic factor deficiencies (see Chapter 52). More recently, greater success has been achieved with the direct infusion of neurotrophic factor into the brain parenchyma rather than using the cerebrospinal fluid (CSF) or periphery, e.g. glial cell line derived neurotrophic factor (GDNF) in Parkinson's disease (see Chapters 39 and 52).

47 Neural plasticity and neurotrophic factors II: The central nervous system

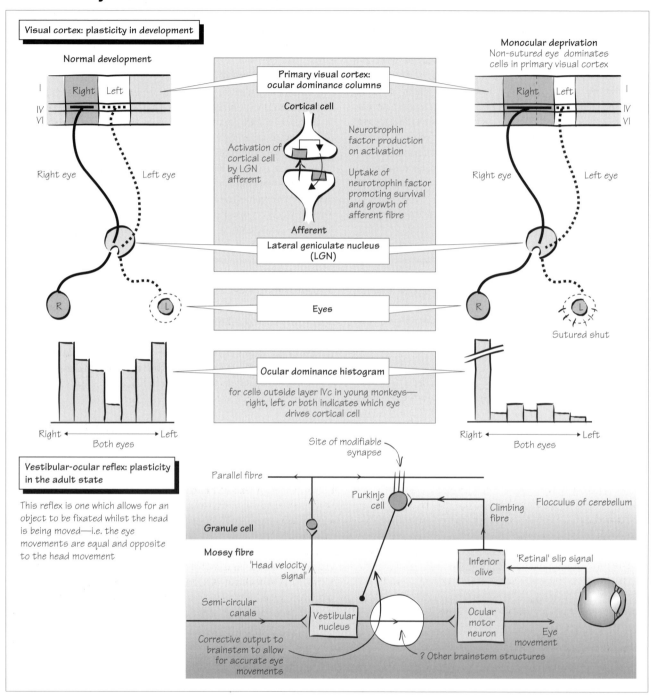

Normal development

Monocular deprivation
Non-sutured eye dominates cells in primary visual cortex

Primary visual cortex: ocular dominance columns

Cortical cell

Activation of cortical cell by LGN afferent

Neurotrophin factor production on activation

Uptake of neurotrophin factor promoting survival and growth of afferent fibre

Afferent

Right eye   Left eye

Right eye   Left eye

Lateral geniculate nucleus (LGN)

Eyes

Sutured shut

Ocular dominance histogram

for cells outside layer IVc in young monkeys—right, left or both indicates which eye drives cortical cell

Right ←→ Left
Both eyes

Right ←→ Left
Both eyes

Vestibular-ocular reflex: plasticity in the adult state

This reflex is one which allows for an object to be fixated whilst the head is being moved—i.e. the eye movements are equal and opposite to the head movement

Site of modifiable synapse

Parallel fibre

Purkinje cell

Climbing fibre

Flocculus of cerebellum

Granule cell

Mossy fibre

'Head velocity signal'

Inferior olive

'Retinal' slip signal

Semi-circular canals

Vestibular nucleus

Ocular motor neuron

Eye movement

Corrective output to brainstem to allow for accurate eye movements

? Other brainstem structures

There is now mounting evidence that regeneration and reorganization can occur in the adult central nervous system (CNS). However, plasticity in the CNS is probably not caused by a major production of new neurones, as most neurones in the mature CNS are postmitotic, but to their ability to extend branching new axons. The time at which this is most florid is in the early postnatal period when the systems of the brain are developing, and it is during this time that major modifications can be made.

The mechanisms underlying this plasticity are not fully known, but the production and uptake of factors promoting neuronal growth and survival (**neurotrophic factors**) are important.

Plasticity in the developing visual system

In their pioneering studies, Hubel and Wiesel demonstrated that at birth the input to laminae IV of the primary visual cortex (V1) is diffuse and that it is only during the **critical period** of development (in cats this is up to 3–14 weeks of postnatal life while in humans it may be several years) that these inputs segregate and form the basis of ocular dominance columns (see Chapter 25).

The segregation of input is dependent on the amount and type of activity within the afferent pathway from each eye; the greater this is, the more likely it is that the afferent input will gain control over those cortical neurones. Thus, ocular dominance (OD) columns will form in the absence of competition between the input from the two eyes but will not develop when there is no afferent input from either eye.

Hubel and Wiesel experimentally manipulated the inputs by initially depriving one eye of an input by suturing it shut (**monocular deprivation**) and then in later experiments by reversing the procedure (**'reverse suturing'**). Monocular deprivation created an expansion of the thalamic influence from the unsutured eye in layer IV with a subsequent shift in OD columns so that more cortical cells were under the control of the open eye. This pattern could be rapidly reversed by 'reverse suturing' during the critical period, which implies that the initial shift in thalamic influence on cortical cells is caused by the activation of synapses that were present but functionally suppressed as there is not enough time for any axonal outgrowth. However, in time the initially suppressed synapses from the uncompetitive eye would be physically lost as the active thalamic input takes over the control of cortical cells.

The correct segregation of the ocular inputs into V1 as OD columns is important for the generation of many of the other visual functions in V1. However, once outside the critical period the ability to modify the visual cortex in such a fashion is reduced, but not lost.

Plasticity in the adult state

Somatosensory system and the vestibulo-ocular reflex

It is now known that the somatosensory system is capable of being remodelled in the face of alterations in the input from the peripheral receptors. Thus, the loss of input from a digit (e.g. by amputation) does not lead to a permanently silent area of cortex, but instead the adjacent cortical areas with sensory inputs from adjacent digits would sprout axons and exert influence over this initially silent cortical area.

Conversely, increased afferent information in a sensory pathway results in an expansion of the cortical area receiving that input. Simplistically, it can be imagined that the activity in a given afferent induces the production of a neurotrophic factor in the postsynaptic cell, which then binds to the appropriate receptor in the active presynaptic terminal promoting its growth and survival. In this way the CNS is constantly remodelling itself based on the amount and type of ongoing afferent information.

Subsequently, it was discovered that major sensory deficits, such as the deafferentation of a whole limb, produced similar results which implied that the reclaiming of cortical areas by adjacent inputs was not solely achieved by the local sprouting of axons in the cortex.

A further example of the plasticity of the mature CNS is seen with the vestibulo-ocular reflex (see Chapters 28 and 37). The vestibular system provides a signal to the CNS on head velocity and this is relayed to the cerebellum via mossy fibres. However, the other input to the cerebellum—the climbing fibre—can provide information on the degree to which the image is slipping across the retina (the degree to which eye movements are compensating for head movement). This input from the climbing fibre is not only important in providing a signal on the degree to which the reflex is working but also provides a critical input to correct it. Thus, if one alters the relationship between ocular and head movements by having the patient wear prisms, for example the reflex adapts with time to compensate for the new relationship and this adaptation is possible because the climbing fibre input can modify the parallel fibre (and so indirectly mossy fibre) input to the Purkinje cell (see Chapter 37). The basis for this latter modification at the level of the Purkinje cell is an intracellular process and is termed **long-term depression** (**LTD**; see Chapter 37).

Neural stem cells

In many adult tissues, cell loss occurring through natural attrition or injury is balanced by the proliferation and subsequent differentiation of stem cells. In the adult CNS this was thought not to be the case, but recent evidence has shown that neural precursor cells are to be found in the mature CNS of mammals including humans. These cells are mainly found in the hippocampus and around the ventricles (in the subventricular zone) and appear to be able to form functionally active neurones. However, their role in plasticity and repair is unknown.

Limits on the regenerative capacity of the adult central nervous system

It must be realized that this regenerative capacity of the CNS is limited as:

1 neurones are postmitotic in the mature CNS, and the stem cell population is small and localized to certain sites; and

2 glial cells in the CNS are generally inhibitory to axonal outgrowth (see Chapter 4).

Astrocytes produce signals that stop axons growing and oligodendrocytes produce a number of factors that repel axons or even cause the approaching axonal growth cone to collapse. This often becomes more apparent at the time of the CNS insult, when glial cells divide, become activated and form a glial scar.

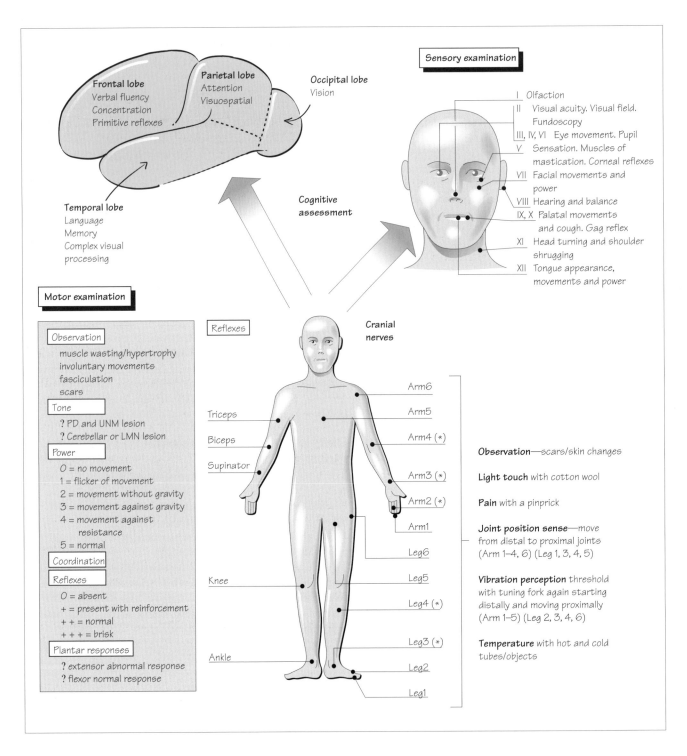

The examination of the nervous system can be broken down into a number of separate assessments.

Cognitive examination
General
Orientation in time, person and place: if this can not be correctly answered (assuming the patient has no major language deficits) then the patient is either acutely confused or severely demented in which case the remainder of the cognitive examination is unlikely to be helpful.

Frontal lobe function
Verbal fluency: number of words generated beginning with a certain letter (e.g. 's') or specific category (e.g. animals) over a 60- or 90-s period.

Concentration: the ability to take in and repeat back immediately a list of objects or a name and address.

Primitive reflexes: including pouting of the lips when they are tapped and grasping the examiner's hand when it is gently moved across the patient's hand.

Parietal lobe function

Attention: or neglect of visual or somatosensory stimuli in the contralateral sensory hemifield.

Dyspraxia: the patient is unable to form, copy or mime gestures and common tasks (e.g. combing hair).

Visuospatial function: the ability to copy drawings.

Temporal lobe function

Anterograde memory: the ability to retain a standard name and address given to the patient (e.g. Peter Marshall, 42 Market Street, Chelmsford, Essex) 5 min after it has been given and retained.

Language: language assessment involves listening to spontaneous speech for content and fluency, naming objects, repeating phrases (e.g. 'no ifs, ands or buts'), following commands, reading and writing.

Cranial nerves

Olfactory nerve: each nostril is tested separately with a range of standard odours.

Optic nerve: visual acuity for each eye is tested using standard eyesight charts. The visual fields for each eye are then tested with examination of the blind spot if necessary (see Chapter 23). The fundi (back of the eye) are examined with an ophthalmoscope looking for abnormalities of the retina and optic disc (e.g. swollen (papilloedema) or pale and atrophic (optic atrophy). Colour vision (using the Ishihara colour plates) and pupillary responses can also be tested.

Oculomotor, trochlear and abducens nerve: ptosis and pupillary abnormalities are looked for (e.g. Horner's syndrome; see Chapter 42). The eye movements in all directions are then tested and the patient reports any diplopia (see Chapter 40).

Trigeminal nerve: sensation is tested in all three divisions of the trigeminal nerve and the power of the jaw muscles. In some cases the corneal reflex is tested by lightly touching the cornea with cotton wool. The patient should respond quickly by rapidly blinking.

Facial nerve: the power of facial muscles is tested, e.g. the patient screws up their eyes tightly, blows out their cheeks or purses their lips. The examiner should *not* be able to overcome any of these movements.

Vestibulocochlear nerve: hearing is tested in each ear by gently whispering a number into each. More formal testing can be performed with tuning forks.

Glossopharyngeal and vagus nerve: the patient opens their mouth wide and says 'ahhhhhh' to assess movement of the palate. The gag reflex can be tested where a spatula is gently placed against the posterior pharyngeal wall and reflex movement of the palate seen. Testing the cough can also be helpful in some cases.

Spinal accessory nerve: tested by getting the patient to turn their head to the right and left and shrug their shoulders. The examiner should not be able to overcome these movements.

Hypoglossal nerve: tested by looking at the tongue in the floor of the mouth for wasting or fasciculation and then it is protruded from the mouth and any deviation from the midline noted. Power is tested by getting the patient to push the tongue into each cheek, assuming they do not have any significant facial weakness.

Motor system examination of the limbs

The examination of the motor system should include the following.

Observation: involuntary movements, wasting, weakness, fasciculation, scars or deformities.

Tone: the limb is gently moved and the stiffness of it assessed. It is increased in Parkinson's disease or upper motorneurone (UMN) lesions and decreased in lower motorneurone (LMN) or cerebellar lesions (see Chapters 32–34). Sometimes the tone is increased because the patient cannot relax.

Power: movements are assessed and scored according to the MRC rating scale (see figure).

Coordination: the ability to coordinate movements in the upper limb is tested by getting the patient to touch the examiner's finger and then their own nose as the finger is slowly moved around in space. This may be abnormal if there is weakness, sensory loss or cerebellar disease. Alternatively, in the upper limb the patient can be asked to rapidly pronate and supinate their hand. In the lower limb coordination is tested by getting the patient to walk normally, then heel–toe walking and finally by getting the patient while lying to run their right/left heel along their left/right shin, respectively.

Reflexes: these are tested by tapping the tendons at certain sites in the upper and lower limb. Reflexes can be absent, reduced, normal or brisk. The latter implies an UMN lesion while reduced or absent reflexes implies a dysfunction in part of the spinal monosynaptic reflex (see Chapter 33).

Plantar responses: the sole of the foot is gently scratched along its lateral aspect and the toes should fan out and the big toe go down (flexor or normal plantar response). If the toes point up and this is not a withdrawal response, then this implies a UMN lesion.

Sensory examination

Sensation in the limbs is tested at the extremities and in the dermatomes using a number of tests.

Light touch: cotton wool is gently applied to the skin, having checked that the patient can feel it normally (test on face first).

Pinprick: using a blunted pin (which is *not* reusable). Do not use needles as these are too sharp.

Temperature: using cold and hot tubes or objects.

Vibration perception threshold (VPT): using a tuning fork applied to the distal interphalangeal joint or big toe. The patient must feel it vibrating and *not* just feel it being applied to the joint. If this is not felt to vibrate, it is moved proximally.

Joint position sense (JPS): tested by slightly moving the terminal joint in the hand or toe, having checked that the patient understands what is meant by up and down movements. This movement should be very slight, as JPS is very sensitive in humans. If the movement cannot be detected then larger movements are made at these joints before moving to more proximal joints, in the same way as for VPT.

49 Investigation of the nervous system

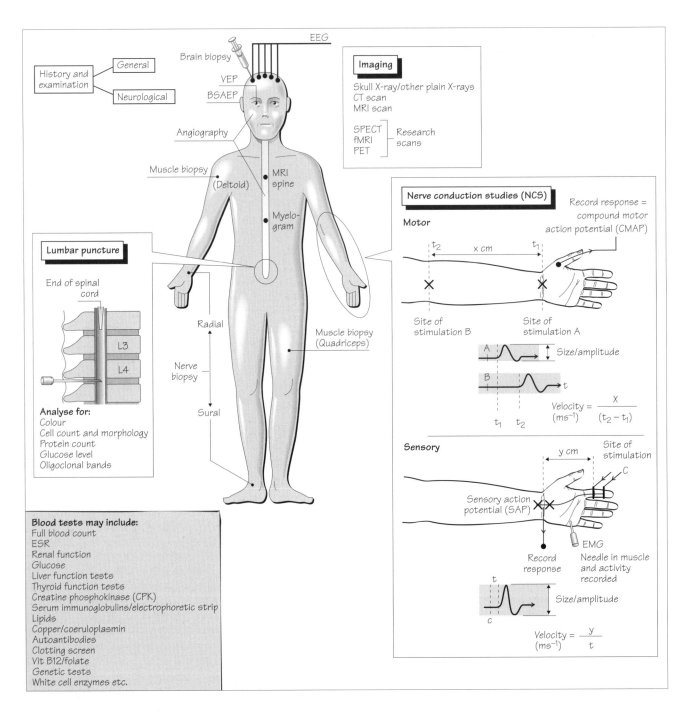

The investigation of the nervous system involves a number of specialist procedures as well as a series of standard tests. However, the key to investigating any patient is through their history and examination, as this will highlight the likely nature and site of the problem. In this chapter the major investigative procedures available in patients with neurological problems are presented, along with their indications.

History and examination

History and examination details the problem, its evolution and other relevant medical history along with the results of the neurological examination (see Chapter 48).

Blood tests

A large number of tests are available (see figure for examples).

Imaging

• Plain X-rays are rarely of value in the diagnosis of neurological disease, unless one suspects the patient has a related disease in another site such as the chest (e.g. lung cancer).

• Computerized tomography (CT) gives detailed X-ray images of the brain, skull and lower spine. It is useful for diagnosing structural lesions such as tumours, major strokes or skull fractures. It is widely available but has limited resolution especially in the posterior fossa and cervicothoracic spinal cord.

• Magnetic resonance imaging (MRI) is a noisy claustrophobic procedure which relies on patient cooperation. It provides detailed images of all parts of the brain and spinal cord and the use of different sequences has increased its utility and diagnostic strength. It does not involve any radiation.

• Magnetic resonance angiography and venography (MRA/MRV) scans delineate the major blood vessels to, within and from the brain. They are primarily used to look for significant narrowing (stenosis) of the extracranial carotid arteries in the neck, aneurysms in the brain and blockage of the major venous sinuses in the brain, but are not as sensitive as angiography.

• Angiography involves the passing of a small catheter to the origin of the major blood vessels of the brain (both carotid and vertebral arteries), and a small amount of dye is injected. The dye can then be followed using a video and images captured rapidly over time as the dye passes through the vascular tree. The procedure is invasive and carries a small risk of complication, but is useful in accurately delineating any vascular abnormality (e.g. carotid stenoses, aneurysms, arteriovenous malformations and venous sinus thrombosis). It can also be used to look for specific vascular abnormalities in the spinal cord.

• Myelography is rarely used nowadays to delineate abnormalities in the spinal cord because of the non-invasiveness and resolution of MRI. However, it can be helpful in some circumstances and involves injecting a radio-opaque dye via a lumbar puncture into the subarachnoid space around the spine.

• Single photon emission computed tomography (SPECT) involves radioactive isotopes which typically provide information on perfusion within the brain. It has low resolution.

• Functional MRI (fMRI) is a research tool that measures activation of specific brain regions by assessing oxygen uptake.

• Positron emission tomography (PET) detects the release of positrons from specific substances which bind to certain chemical sites within the brain. It is only used for research purposes.

Electrical tests

• Electrocardiography (ECG) is an electrical recording from the heart, and is performed in many patients with neurological disease, especially those with muscle disease, blackouts or some genetic disorders.

• Electroencephalography (EEG) measures the electrical activity and rhythms of the brain and is helpful in patients with decreased levels of consciousness and epilepsy.

• Nerve conduction studies (NCS) involve stimulating both sensory and motor nerves and measuring the response. The general principle is that one stimulates at one site of the nerve and records at another or the muscle it innervates. The size and speed of the response are important. Loss of myelin (demyelination) slows the speed of conduction, while a loss of axons gives a smaller response but normal conduction velocity. It is useful in determining whether the patient has a neuropathy, what type (demyelinating vs. axonal) and the extent (focal or generalized).

• Electromyography (EMG) involves placing a needle into the muscle and recording the electrical activity within it. It is useful in the diagnosis of muscle disease.

• Evoked potentials (EPs) can be in the visual pathway (visual-evoked potential or responses; VEP), auditory pathway (brainstem auditory-evoked potential) or peripheral nerves in the arms or legs (somatosensory-evoked potential). The test involves stimulating the peripheral receptor (eye, ear or median/posterior tibial nerve) and measuring the cortical response. This gives a measure of conduction along the pathway that has both a peripheral and CNS component. The most commonly used test is VEP in *multiple sclerosis* looking for asymptomatic demyelination in the visual pathways.

• Central motor conduction time (CMCT) measures the time from stimulating the motor cortex to measuring a muscle response in the periphery such as the hand. It is not routinely available and is a measure of integrity of the descending corticospinal tract.

• Thermal thresholds is a subjective test designed to look at small fibre responses in patients. It relies on the patient detecting changes in temperature in the hands and feet. It is not routinely available in most centres.

Cerebrospinal fluid analysis

Cerebrospinal fluid (CSF) can be obtained from a number of sites but is routinely obtained by a lumbar puncture, which involves passing a small needle into the subarachnoid space in the lower lumbar spine. CSF should be clear and the opening pressure is measured before three separate tubes of fluid are sent for analysis including the following.

• Number and type of cells, typically raised in infections such as meningitis.

• Culture of the CSF to look for infective organisms, including a Gram stain in meningitis.

• Glucose, which can be low in certain types of infection/meningitis and metastatic tumours growing in the meninges.

• Protein, which can be raised in some types of neuropathy, tumour and in lesions causing a block to spinal CSF flow.

• Oligoclonal bands indicative of immunoglobulin synthesis within the CNS, typically seen in multiple sclerosis.

Nerve/muscle biopsy

In cases where there is evidence of nerve or muscle disease, a biopsy may be helpful in identifying the defect more specifically. Typical sites are the radial and sural nerves and the quadriceps and deltoid muscles.

Brain biopsy

This is routinely performed in patients with brain tumours to confirm the diagnosis and to some extent predict prognosis. In some cases of progressive neurological disease for which no obvious cause can be found, a biopsy looking specifically for inflammation in the blood vessels (vasculitis) as well as prion disease may be considered. However, in the latter case, strict guidelines must be followed with respect to the reuse/disposal of the instruments.

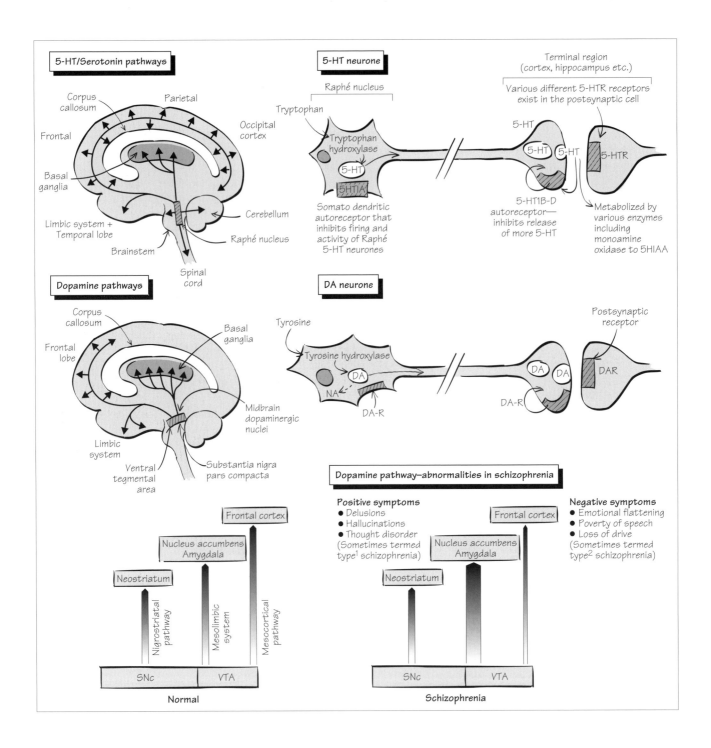

There are a large number of psychiatric disorders that have many causes and treatments including affective disorders or disorders of mood such as *depression* and *mania* (when the mood oscillates between depression and mania it is termed a bipolar disorder). Depression is characterized by sadness, apathy, low self-esteem and a tendency to withdraw from others coupled to a loss of libido, anorexia and early morning waking. Mania, on the other hand, is characterized by euphoria, delusions of grandeur and mental overactivity.

Schizophrenia is a syndrome characterized by specific psychological manifestations, including auditory hallucinations, delusions, thought disorders and behavioural disturbances.

Depression

The cause of endogenous depression is not known, but although there is clearly a genetic component to the disorder, the nature of this is unclear.

A number of different therapies are employed for the treatment of depression, and while these include psychotherapy and electroconvulsive therapy (ECT), the most commonly used approach is with antidepressant drugs. Most of the drugs in the treatment of depression inhibit the reuptake of noradrenaline (norepinephrine) and/or serotonin (5-HT). Less commonly used drugs are inhibitors of monoamine oxidase (MAOIs). Because both uptake inhibitors and MAOIs increase the amount of noradrenaline (norepinephrine) and/or 5-HT in the synaptic cleft and so enhance the action of these transmitters, it was argued that depression resulted from an 'underactivity' of these monoaminergic systems. This simple idea is often referred to as the monoamine theory of depression and is a useful hypothesis, although not an entirely adequate explanation for this condition.

Amine uptake inhibitors

Tricyclic antidepressants (e.g. imipramine, amitriptyline) have proven antidepressant actions but no one drug has greater efficacy. Some have sedative actions (e.g. amitriptyline) and are more useful for agitated and anxious patients (see Chapter 51).

Drugs that are specific serotonin reuptake inhibitors (SSRIs, e.g. fluoxetine) do not have the troublesome autonomic side-effects of the tricyclics but may cause nausea and gastrointestinal problems.

Monoamine oxidase inhibitors

The older MAOIs (e.g. phenelzine) are irreversible non-selective inhibitors of MAO. Their efficacy is similar to the tricyclics but unwanted side-effects (e.g. postural hypotension) and potentially serious interaction with foods containing tyramine have limited their use. Moclobemide is a newer drug that selectively inhibits MAO_A and lacks most of the unwanted effects of phenelzine.

Schizophrenia

Schizophrenia has a significant genetic component, with the risk for a first-degree relative developing the disease of 10%, rising to 40% for the offspring if both parents are affected.

Early theories of schizophrenia proposed that it was caused by the production of some endogenous psychotogen that may be a trans-methylated derivative of dopamine. Subsequently, this was modified to the theory that schizophrenia was caused by overactivity of the central dopaminergic pathways, especially the mesolimbic projections with relative sparing of the dopaminergic nigrostriatal pathway (see Chapter 38).

This has been further modified to the theory that the negative symptoms of schizophrenia may be caused by hypodopaminergic activity in the mesocortical system, while the psychotic symptoms result from hyperdopaminergic activity in the mesolimbic system. Indeed, schizophrenics show frontal hypoperfusion and this, coupled to previous studies showing non-progressive cerebral ventricular dilatation without gliosis, led to the proposal that schizophrenia may be a neurodevelopmental disorder. However, which part of the brain fails to develop normally is not known, although the amygdala, frontal and temporal lobes seem likely candidates.

The mainstay of therapy in schizophrenia remains the use of drugs that block the dopamine receptors, of which there are least five subtypes (D_1–D_5 receptors; see Appendix 1). These agents (e.g. chlorpromazine) are called antipsychotics or neuroleptics. It is not known how these agents reduce the severity of the symptoms in schizophrenia. A correlation between the clinical dose of antipsychotic drugs and their affinity to D_2 receptors suggests that blockade of this receptor subtype may be particularly important.

Antipsychotic drugs require several weeks to control the symptoms of schizophrenia and most patients require maintenance treatment for many years. Relapses are common even in drug-maintained patients. Unfortunately, neuroleptics also block dopamine (DA) receptors in the basal ganglia, often producing distressing and disabling movement disorders (e.g. **Parkinsonism**; see Chapter 39). Blockade of D_2 receptors in the pituitary gland causes an increase in prolactin release and endocrine effects (e.g. gynaecomastia, galactorrhoea; see Chapter 43). Many neuroleptics also block muscarinic receptors (causing dry mouth, blurred vision, constipation), α-adrenoceptors (postural hypotension) and histamine H_1 receptors (sedation).

Some newer drugs ('atypical' agents) have a reduced tendency to cause movement disorders (e.g. clozapine, risperidone, olanzapine) but the reason for this is unknown. Clozapine is restricted to patients resistant to other drugs because it causes neutropenia or agranulocytosis in about 4% of patients. Risperidone and other newer atypical agents are increasingly used in the treatment of schizophrenia because they are more acceptable to patients.

51 Neurochemical disorders II: Anxiety

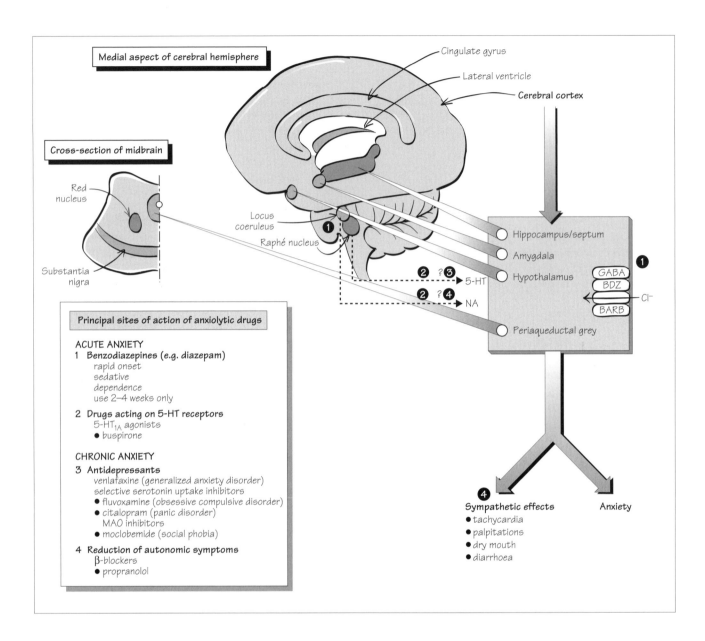

Medial aspect of cerebral hemisphere

Cingulate gyrus
Lateral ventricle
Cerebral cortex

Cross-section of midbrain

Red nucleus
Locus coeruleus
Raphé nucleus
Substantia nigra

Hippocampus/septum
Amygdala
Hypothalamus
Periaqueductal grey

GABA
BDZ
BARB
Cl⁻

5-HT
NA

Principal sites of action of anxiolytic drugs

ACUTE ANXIETY
1 Benzodiazepines (e.g. diazepam)
   rapid onset
   sedative
   dependence
   use 2–4 weeks only

2 Drugs acting on 5-HT receptors
   5-HT$_{1A}$ agonists
   • buspirone

CHRONIC ANXIETY
3 Antidepressants
   venlafaxine (generalized anxiety disorder)
   selective serotonin uptake inhibitors
   • fluvoxamine (obsessive compulsive disorder)
   • citalopram (panic disorder)
     MAO inhibitors
   • moclobemide (social phobia)

4 Reduction of autonomic symptoms
   β-blockers
   • propranolol

Sympathetic effects
• tachycardia
• palpitations
• dry mouth
• diarrhoea

Anxiety

Anxiety is a normal emotional reaction to threatening or potentially threatening situations, and is accompanied by sympathetic overactivity. In **anxiety disorders** the patient experiences anxiety that is disproportionate to the stimulus, and sometimes in the absence of any obvious stimulus. There is no organic basis for anxiety disorders, the symptoms resulting from overactivity of the brain areas involved in 'normal' anxiety. Psychiatric disorders that occur without any known brain pathology are called **neuroses**.

Anxiety disorders are subdivided into four main types: *generalized anxiety disorder*, *panic disorder*, *stress reactions* and *phobias*. Many transmitters seem to be involved in the neural mechanisms of anxiety, the evidence being especially strong for **γ-aminobutyric acid (GABA)** and **5-hydroxytryptamine (5-HT)**. Because intravenous injections of **cholecystokinin (CCK$_4$)** into humans cause the symptoms of panic it has been suggested that abnormalities in different transmitter systems

might be involved in particular types of anxiety disorder. This remains to be seen.

Treatment of mild anxiety disorders may only require simple *supportive psychotherapy*, but in severe anxiety anxiolytic drugs given for a short period are useful. The **benzodiazepines** (e.g. *diazepam*) produce their effects by enhancing GABA-mediated inhibition (see Chapter 53) in many of the brain areas involved in anxiety, including the raphe nucleus (RN). **Tricyclic antidepressants** (e.g. *amitriptyline*) have anxiolytic activity but the mechanism involved is unknown. **β-adrenoceptor antagonists** have a limited use in the treatment of situational anxiety (e.g. in musicians) where palpitations and tremor are the main symptoms. Efforts to discover non-sedative anxiolytics have led to the trial of several drugs that act on specific 5-HT receptors. They have not been very successful.

Anxiety disorders

Generalized anxiety disorders have both psychological and physical symptoms. The psychological symptoms include a feeling of fearful anticipation, difficulty in concentrating, irritability and repetitive worrying thoughts that are often linked to awareness of sympathetic overactivity.

Phobic anxiety disorders have the same core symptoms as generalized anxiety disorders but occur only under certain circumstances, e.g. the appearance of a spider (arachnophobia). In contrast, **panic attacks** are episodic attacks of anxiety in which physical symptoms predominate (e.g. choking, palpitations, chest pain, sweating, trembling).

Benzodiazepines

Benzodiazepines (e.g. diazepam) are central depressants that induce sleep when given in high doses at night and provide sedation and reduce anxiety when given in divided doses during the day. The benzodiazepines are discussed in more detail in Chapter 53, and their main adverse effects are drowsiness, impaired alertness, agitation and ataxia. In anxiety disorders, benzodiazepines should only be given for a maximum of 2–3 weeks because longer treatment risks the development of **dependence**. If this occurs, stopping the drug frequently leads to a **withdrawal syndrome** characterized by anxiety, tremor, sweating and insomnia—symptoms similar to the original complaint.

Sites of action of benzodiazepines in the brain

The areas of the brain involved in the anxiolytic action of the benzodiazepines have been studied in rats by injecting tiny quantities of a drug through cannulae implanted in different brain areas. In general, limbic and brainstem structures seem important in mediating the anxiolytic actions of these drugs. In humans, cerebral blood flow and glucose metabolism studies using positron emission tomography (PET) have not revealed consistent differences in anxious and non-anxious subjects.

Serotonin

Serotonin (5-HT) cell bodies are located in the raphe nuclei of the mid-brain and project to many areas of the brain including those thought to be important in anxiety (hippocampus, amygdala, frontal cortex; see Chapter 50). In rats, lesions of the raphe nuclei produce anxiolytic effects, while stimulation of 5-HT_{1A} autoreceptors with agonists such as 8-hydroxy-DPAT produce anxiogenic effects. A role for 5-HT in anxiety was strengthened when it was found that benzodiazepines reduce the turnover of 5-HT in the brain, and when microinjected into the raphe nucleus, reduce the rate of neuronal firing and produce an anxiolytic effect. However, stimulation of postsynaptic 5-HT_{1A} receptors in limbic areas has anxiogenic effects. These opposing pre- and post-synaptic actions may explain why buspirone, a 5-HT_{1A} partial agonist, has limited efficacy and works after only several weeks. Specific antagonists at 5-HT_3 receptors (e.g. ondansetron) and 5-HT_2 receptors (e.g. ritanserin) have little, if any, anxiolytic actions in humans.

Noradrenaline (norepinephrine)

The evidence for the role of noradrenaline (norepinephrine) in anxiety is much less compelling than that for GABA and 5-HT. Nevertheless, β-adrenoceptor antagonists have a limited use in the treatment of patients with mild or transient anxiety and where autonomic symptoms such as palpitations and tremor are the most troublesome symptoms. The beneficial effects of β-blockers in these patients may result from a peripheral action because those (e.g. practolol) that do not pass the blood–brain barrier are equally effective.

Peptides

Several neuropeptides have been implicated in anxiety. The strongest evidence is for the anxiogenic effect of corticotrophin releasing hormone (CRH), and CRH has also been implicated in depression. Substance P may also have anxiogenic effects and a NK_1 receptor antagonist is in clinical trials for anxiety and depression. CCK is a gut peptide that also occurs in the brain. Because CCK_4 is one of the few agents (CO_2 is another) that elicits genuine panic-like attacks, it was hoped that CCK antagonists would be useful anxiolytics, but so far no useful drug has emerged.

52 Neurodegenerative disorders

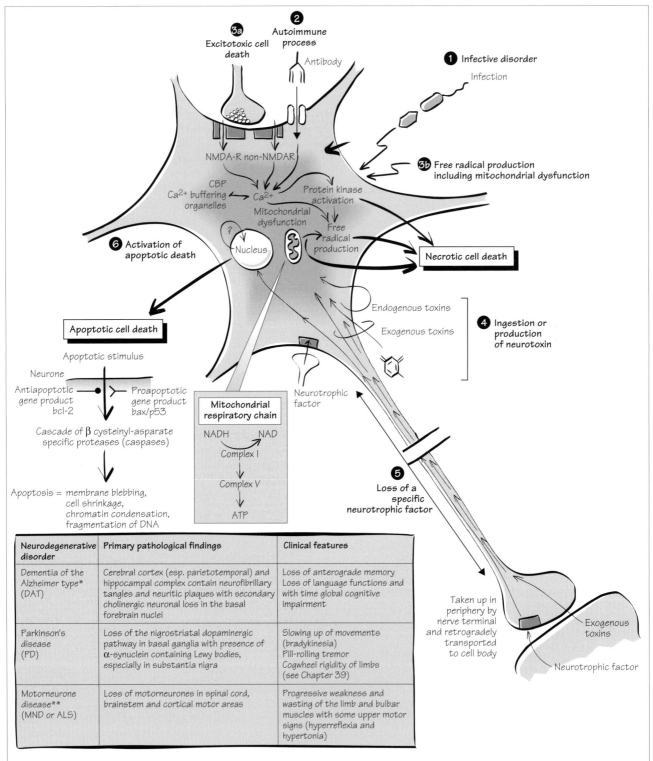

Neurodegenerative disorder	Primary pathological findings	Clinical features
Dementia of the Alzheimer type* (DAT)	Cerebral cortex (esp. parietotemporal) and hippocampal complex contain neurofibrillary tangles and neuritic plaques with secondary cholinergic neuronal loss in the basal forebrain nuclei	Loss of anterograde memory Loss of language functions and with time global cognitive impairment
Parkinson's disease (PD)	Loss of the nigrostriatal dopaminergic pathway in basal ganglia with presence of α-synuclein containing Lewy bodies, especially in substantia nigra	Slowing up of movements (bradykinesia) Pill-rolling tremor Cogwheel rigidity of limbs (see Chapter 39)
Motorneurone disease** (MND or ALS)	Loss of motorneurones in spinal cord, brainstem and cortical motor areas	Progressive weakness and wasting of the limb and bulbar muscles with some upper motor signs (hyperreflexia and hypertonia)

* Some forms of dementia have a more focal onset with selective involvement of the frontotemporal cortex, some cases of which have cortical inclusion (Pick) bodies at autopsy. These disorders are commonly termed fronto temporal dementia

** Motorneurone disease can present with either purely LMN or UMN features, but the commonest presentation is with a combination of the two —a condition also known as amyotrophic lateral sclerosis or ALS

NB A range of other neurodegenerative disorders are not discussed in this chapter and include Huntington's disease (Chapters 39 and 55) and spinocerebellar degenerations (Chapter 55). The mechanisms of cell death in these conditions may be similar to those described in this chapter

Neurodegenerative disorders are those conditions in which the primary pathological event is a progressive loss of specific populations of central nervous system (CNS) neurones over time.

Aetiology of neurodegenerative disorders

There are a number of theories on the aetiology of neurodegenerative disorders which may not be mutually exclusive.

1 An infective disorder

Neuronal death with a glial reaction (gliosis) is commonly seen in infective disorders (typically viral) with inflammation in the CNS. However, in neurodegenerative disorders such a reaction is not seen, although the observation that *HIV infection* can cause a dementia has raised the possibility that some neurodegenerative disorders may be caused by a retroviral infection. Furthermore, the development of dementia with spongiform changes throughout the brain in response to the proliferation of abnormal prion proteins as occurs in *Creutzfeldt–Jakob disease* has further fuelled the debate on an infective aetiology in some neurodegenerative disorders.

2 An autoimmune process

Autoantibodies have been described in some neurodegenerative conditions, e.g. antibodies to calcium channels in *motorneurone disease (MND)*. However, the absence of an inflammatory response would argue against this hypothesis, although neuronal degeneration with a minimal inflammatory infiltrate can be seen in the *paraneoplastic syndromes* (see Chapter 54).

3 The result of excitotoxic cell death and free radical production

Excitatory amino acids are found throughout the CNS (see Chapter 9) and act on a range of receptors that serve to depolarize the neurone and allow Ca^{2+} to influx into the cell. On entering the neurone calcium is normally quickly buffered; if the level of excitation is great then there may be an excessive influx of Ca^{2+} which can lead to the production of toxic free radicals and cell death. It is this cascade of events that may underlie some of the neurodegenerative disorders. For example, in some cases of familial *MND* there is a loss of one of the free radical scavenger molecules—superoxide dismutase. Furthermore, in Parkinson's disease, deficiency in complex I activity of the mitochondrial respiratory chain in the substantia nigra may lead to the overproduction of free radicals as well as compromised cellular respiration—both of which contribute to neuronal death.

4 The ingestion or production of a neurotoxin

Many toxins can induce degenerative conditions (e.g. parkinsonism with manganese poisoning) but no such exogenous compound has consistently been found to cause any of the major neurodegenerative disorders.

Dementia of the Alzheimer type (DAT), on the other hand, is associated with the development of neurofibrillary tangles (NFTs) and senile neuritic plaques (SNPs) in the parahippocampal and parietotemporal cortical areas. The density of NFTs correlates well with the cognitive state of the patient. NFTs contain paired helical filaments made up of an abnormal form of the microtubule-associated protein τ—a protein that normally serves to maintain the neuronal cytoskeleton. In contrast, SNPs contain abnormal forms of the protein β-amyloid, derived from the membrane-bound glycoprotein amyloid precursor protein (APP) which is found in all neurones in normal brains and which performs some unknown function.

The reason as to why these abnormal proteins are produced and in what order is not clear—certainly some of the rare familial forms of **DAT** have genetic defects that influence the production of the amyloid protein. Whatever the reason for the development of these abnormal proteins, the result is cell death within the cortex. This leads to a secondary loss in the cholinergic innervation of the cortex with an associated atrophy of the cholinergic neurones in the basal forebrain, which has prompted clinical studies in the use of drugs that potentiate CNS cholinergic transmission, although these have met with only limited success. In addition, a range of neurodegenerative disorders have now been found to contain intracellular inclusions of abnormal protein (e.g. huntingtin in Huntington's disease, τ in some complex parkinsonian conditions, α-synuclein in Parkinson's disease), and thus some common pathogenic cellular pathway may underlie the actual loss of neurones in all these conditions.

5 The loss of a specific neurotrophic factor

Neurones are maintained by the production of a specific growth or neurotrophic factor (see Chapters 46 and 47), and the loss of one or some of these factors may underlie the development of the various neurodegenerative disorders. Clinical trials using neurotrophic factors in patients with neurodegenerative disorders have been undertaken with some recent success with glial cell line derived neurotrophic factor (GDNF) and Parkinson's disease.

6 The activation of a cell death programme (apoptosis)

The loss of cells in most conditions (e.g. inflammation) is by a process of necrotic cell death but all cells contain the necessary machinery to initiate their own death: programmed cell death or apoptosis. The pathways underlying this process are now relatively well understood although the triggers initiating them are not clear. It is therefore possible that neurodegenerative disorders are caused by an inappropriate activation of this programme, possibly secondary to the loss of a neurotrophic factor.

53 Neurophysiological disorders: epilepsy

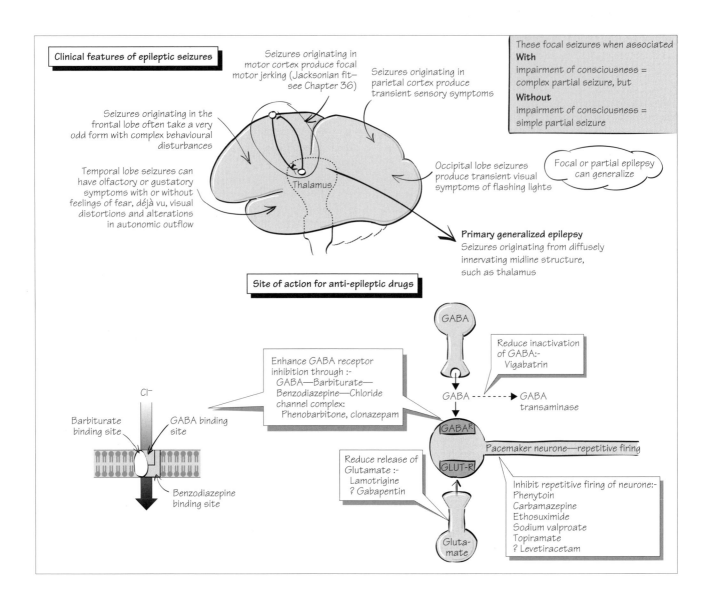

Definition and classification of epilepsy

Epilepsy represents a transitory disturbance of the functions of the brain that develops suddenly, ceases spontaneously and may be induced by a number of different provocations. It is the most prevalent serious neurological condition with a peak incidence in early childhood and in the elderly.

Patients with epileptic fits or seizures may be classified according to whether the fit is **generalized** or **partial (focal)**, i.e. remains within one small central nervous system (CNS) site, e.g. temporal lobe; whether there is an impairment of consciousness (if there is then it is termed **complex**); or whether the partial seizure causes secondary generalization. Overall, 60–70% of all epileptics have no obvious cause for their seizures, and about two-thirds of all patients stop having seizures within 2–5 years of their onset, usually in the context of taking medication.

Pathogenesis of epilepsy

The **aetiology of epilepsy** is largely unknown, but much of the therapy used to treat this condition works by modifying either the balance between the inhibitory γ-aminobutyric acid (GABA) and excitatory glutamatergic networks within the brain or the repetitive firing potential of neurones. The recording of the electroencephalograph (EEG; see Chapters 44 and 49) reveals that **epileptic fits** (ictal events) are associated with either generalized synchronous or focal spike and wave discharges, although abnormalities can be seen transiently at other times without overt evidence of a seizure (**interictal activity**).

A generalized epileptic fit can take several forms but classically consists of a tonic (muscles go stiff)–clonic (jerking of limbs and body) phase followed by a period of unconsciousness. This used to be termed a grand mal seizure, but is now classified as a generalized tonic–clonic seizure. Petit mal epilepsy is now reclassified as a form of primary generalized epilepsy.

A model for the generation of an epileptic discharge is that the interictal activity corresponds to a depolarizing shift with superimposed action potentials from an assembly of neurones. There follows a period of hyperpolarization as these same neurones activate local inhibitory interneurones while becoming inactivated themselves.

With repeated interictal spikes the period of hyperpolarization shortens and this activates a range of normally quiescent ion channels in the neurone as well as raising extracellular K^+ concentrations, all of which further depolarizes the neurones. If sufficient neurones are activated (and the inhibition of local GABA interneurones overcome) then synchronous discharges are produced across populations of neurones which can lead on to a seizure. The seizure or synchronous discharge is then terminated by active processes of inhibition both within the neurone (through ion channels) and within the neuronal network by GABAergic interneuronal activity.

Although this model is useful as a means of understanding the cellular physiology of epilepsy irrespective of cause, it is clear that different forms of epilepsy have different underlying abnormalities. *Primary generalized epilepsy*, which is associated with diffuse EEG changes, is thought to result from abnormalities in specific calcium channels in the thalamus. Patients with *complex partial seizures of temporal lobe origin* may have a small scar in the mesial temporal lobe corresponding to neuronal loss and gliosis within the hippocampus, secondary to hypoxic or ischaemic insults early in life.

Treatment of epilepsy

The treatment of epilepsy involves drug therapy or a surgical approach if an underlying structural lesion is identified and/or drug therapy is ineffective. Drug therapy is useful in all forms of epilepsy. Administration of a single drug will control the fits in 70–80% of patients with tonic–clonic seizures and 30–40% of patients with partial seizures. Poorly controlled patients may benefit from the addition of a second 'add-on' drug but only about 7% of the refractory patients become completely seizure free.

Mechanisms of action of antiepileptic drugs

These are not well understood. Some drugs (e.g. benzodiazepines, vigabatrin, phenobarbital) enhance GABA-mediated inhibition, while others are Na^+-channel blockers (phenytoin, carbamazepine, sodium valproate, lamotrigine). Ethosuximide, which is effective only in absences, inhibits the spike-generating Ca^{2+} current in thalamic neu-

rones. Sodium valproate also has this action on Ca^{2+} channels in addition to its effects on Na^+ channels, explaining its wide-spectrum of anticonvulsant action.

Carbamazepine, sodium valproate and lamotrigine are widely used because of their efficacy and well-documented but largely tolerable side-effects.

The advantages of **sodium valproate** are its relative lack of sedative effects, its wide spectrum of activity and the mild nature of its adverse effects (nausea, weight gain, bleeding tendencies, tremor and transient hair loss). The main disadvantage is that occasional idiosyncratic responses cause severe or fatal hepatic toxicity and teratogenicity. For this reason, **carbamazepine** or lamotrigine is often preferred. Mild neurotoxic effects are common (nausea, headache, drowsiness, diplopia and ataxia) and often determine the limit of dosage. Agranulocytosis is a rare idiosyncratic reaction to carbamazepine. **Lamotrigine** is a relatively new drug with a broad range of efficacy and is especially safe in pregnancy. **Phenytoin** is a difficult drug to use because of its complex metabolism, such that it may take up to 20 days for the serum level to stabilize after changing the dose. Therefore, the dose must be increased gradually until fits are prevented, or until signs of *cerebellar disturbance* occur (nystagmus, ataxia, dysarthia). Other unpleasant side-effects, including gum hypertrophy, acne, greasy skin, coarsening of the facial features and hirsuitism, make the drug unpopular with patients, especially women. **Phenobarbital** is effective in tonic–clonic and partial seizures but is very sedative. Tolerance occurs and sudden withdrawal may precipitate status epilepticus. Side-effects include *cerebellar symptoms*, drowsiness in adults and hyperkinesia in children. **Vigabatrin, gabapentin, topiramate** and **levetiracetam** are newer agents introduced as 'add-on' drugs in patients where epilepsy is not satisfactorily controlled by other antiepileptics. **Ethosuximide** is only effective in the treatment of absences and myoclonic seizures (brief jerky movements without loss of consciousness). **Clonazepam** is a potent benzodiazepine anticonvulsant that is effective in absences, tonic–clonic seizures and myoclonic seizures. It is very sedative and tolerance occurs with prolonged oral administration.

Anticonvulsant therapy in pregnancy requires care because of the teratogenic potential of many of these drugs, especially valproate and phenytoin.

54 Neuroimmunological disorders

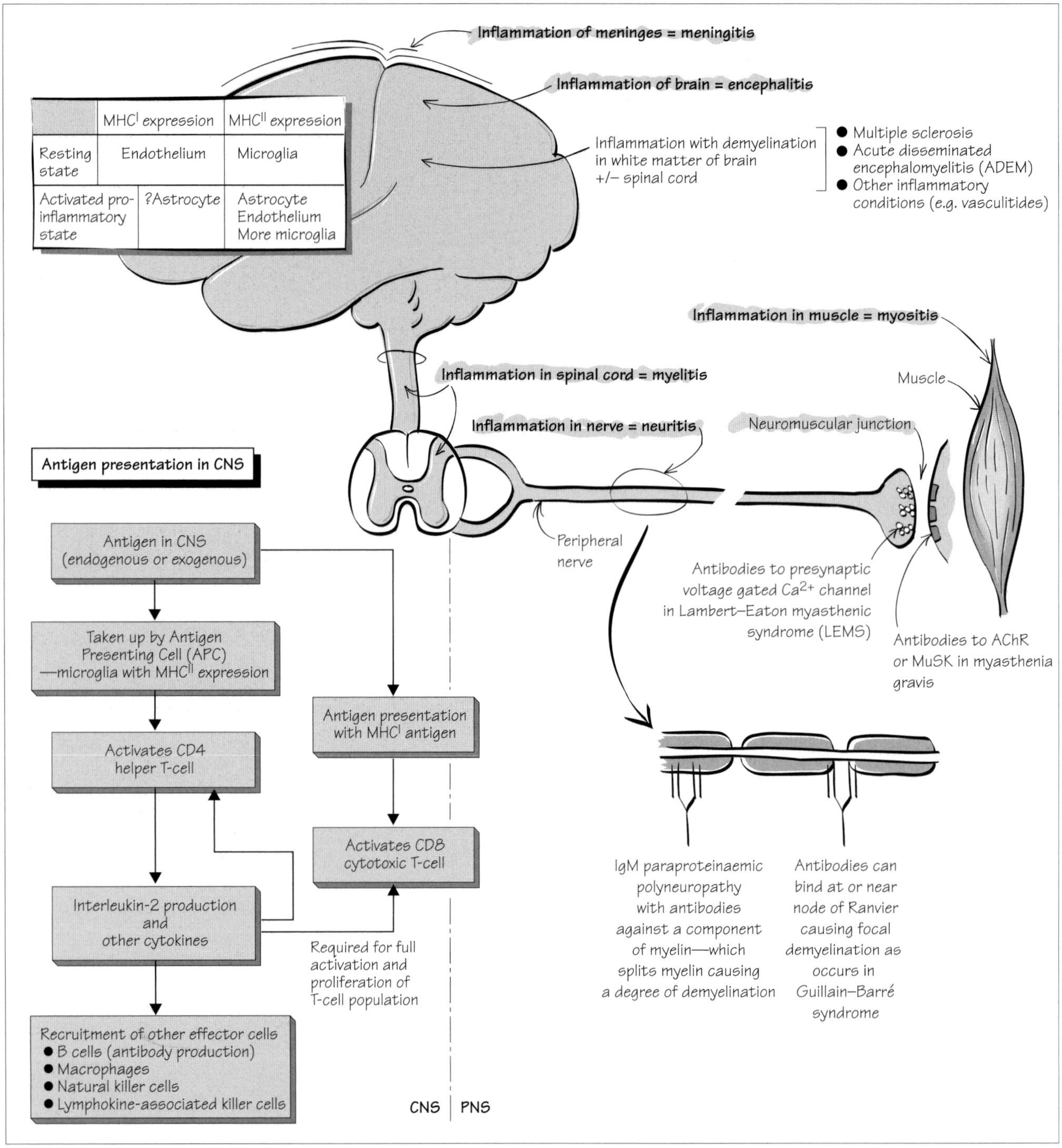

Inflammation of meninges = meningitis
Inflammation of brain = encephalitis
MHC^{I} expression
MHC^{II} expression
Resting state
Endothelium
Microglia
Activated pro-inflammatory state
?Astrocyte
Astrocyte Endothelium More microglia
Inflammation with demyelination in white matter of brain +/– spinal cord
● Multiple sclerosis
● Acute disseminated encephalomyelitis (ADEM)
● Other inflammatory conditions (e.g. vasculitides)
Inflammation in muscle = myositis
Inflammation in spinal cord = myelitis
Muscle
Inflammation in nerve = neuritis
Neuromuscular junction
Antigen presentation in CNS
Antigen in CNS (endogenous or exogenous)
Taken up by Antigen Presenting Cell (APC) —microglia with MHC^{II} expression
Activates CD4 helper T-cell
Antigen presentation with MHC^{I} antigen
Activates CD8 cytotoxic T-cell
Interleukin-2 production and other cytokines
Required for full activation and proliferation of T-cell population
Recruitment of other effector cells
● B cells (antibody production)
● Macrophages
● Natural killer cells
● Lymphokine-associated killer cells
CNS
PNS
Peripheral nerve
Antibodies to presynaptic voltage gated Ca^{2+} channel in Lambert–Eaton myasthenic syndrome (LEMS)
Antibodies to AChR or MuSK in myasthenia gravis
IgM paraproteinaemic polyneuropathy with antibodies against a component of myelin—which splits myelin causing a degree of demyelination
Antibodies can bind at or near node of Ranvier causing focal demyelination as occurs in Guillain–Barré syndrome

Central nervous system immunological network

The central nervous system (CNS) has relative **immunological privilege** compared with the peripheral nervous system (PNS) and most other parts of the body. The reason for this is that the **blood–brain barrier (BBB)** normally prevents most lymphocytes, macrophages and antibodies from entering the CNS (see Chapters 4 and 16). This, coupled to the very poorly developed lymphatic drainage system of the CNS and the low level of expression of major histocompatibility complex (MHC) antigens means that antigen presentation is poor. However, breakdown of the BBB can greatly alter this situation.

In the resting state some activated T-lymphocytes are able to cross the BBB and circulate within the CNS. In addition, **MHC expression** is confined to only a few cells although the situation is different in the inflamed state. Thus, once triggered an immune response can be amplified and propagated by the elaboration of cytokines and induced MHC expression with the opening up of the BBB.

In these circumstances the **microglia** are thought to be important as the **antigen presenting cells** and their interaction with T-helper lymphocytes is then pivotal in generating a full-blown immunological reaction.

Clinical disorders of the central nervous system with an immunological basis

Multiple sclerosis

Multiple sclerosis is a common neurological disorder in which the patient characteristically presents with episodes of neurological dysfunction secondary to inflammatory lesions within the CNS. Pathologically, these lesions represent small areas of demyelination secondary to an underlying inflammatory (mainly T-cell) infiltrate — the trigger and target for which is not clear. The lesions often resolve with remyelination and clinical recovery, although with time a permanent loss of myelin ensues with secondary axonal loss and the development of fixed disabilities.

To date the most successful therapies are high-dose intravenous methylprednisolone which hastens recovery from acute relapses but does not alter the long-term disease process, and β-interferon which reduces the relapse rate but again has, as yet, an unproven role in modifying the long-term prognosis. More aggressive immunotherapy with drugs such as CAMPATH may prove to be more effective, especially if given early on in the course of the disease.

Acute disseminated encephalomyelitis

This is a rare inflammatory demyelinating disease of the CNS that occurs as a complication of a number of infections and vaccinations (e.g. measles and rabies vaccination). It is a monophasic illness (unlike multiple sclerosis) characterized by widespread disseminated lesions throughout the CNS that pathologically consist of an intense perivascular infiltrate of lymphocytes and macrophages with demyelination. This condition resembles **experimental allergic encephalomyelitis** which is a well-characterized T-cell mediated disorder against a component of myelin (probably myelin basic protein) induced by inoculating animals with a combination of sterile brain tissue and adjuvants.

Other immunological diseases

A number of other diseases with an immunological basis can affect the CNS and these include those diseases that primarily affect blood vessels (the *vasculitides*).

In addition, there is a rare group of disorders in which there is CNS dysfunction as a remote effect of a cancer, *paraneoplastic syndromes*. In these conditions antibodies to components of the CNS are generated, presumably triggered by the tumour, which then lead to neuronal cell death and the development of a neurological syndrome, e.g. anti-Purkinje cell antibodies cause a profound cerebellar syndrome by the immunological removal of this cell type in the cerebellum. The exact mechanism by which these antibodies exert their effect is not known as antibodies normally do not cross the BBB, but pathologically there is often evidence of a lymphocytic infiltrate in the affected structure which implies that the antibody is capable of inducing an immune-mediated process of neuronal loss.

Clinical disorders of the peripheral nervous system with an immunological basis

The PNS has fewer of the protective features of the CNS so is more susceptible to conventional immune-mediated diseases.

• The **peripheral nerve** is affected by a number of immunological processes, including *Guillain–Barré syndrome*. In this condition there is often a preceding illness (e.g. *Campylobacter jejuni* or cytomegalovirus infection) that induces an immune response which then cross-reacts with components in the peripheral nerve (e.g. certain gangliosides). This then induces focal demyelination in the peripheral nerve, which prevents it from conducting action potentials normally (see Chapter 6). In time the patient usually recovers although they may require immunotherapy with either plasma exchange or intravenous immunoglobulin. A similar condition is seen in some diseases where abnormal amounts of a component of antibodies is produced (the *paraproteinaemias*).

• The **neuromuscular junction** can be affected by immunological processes as occurs in *myasthenia gravis* and the *Lambert–Eaton myasthenic syndrome* (see Chapter 7).

• **Muscles** can be involved in inflammatory processes. The most common form of this is *polymyositis*, which is a T-cell mediated condition associated with proximal weakness and pain. In contrast, *dermatomyositis* is a B-cell mediated disease centred on blood vessels which causes a painful proximal muscle weakness in association with a florid skin rash. This latter condition can represent a paraneoplastic syndrome in more elderly patients with tumours in the lung, breast, colon or ovary.

55 Neurogenetic disorders

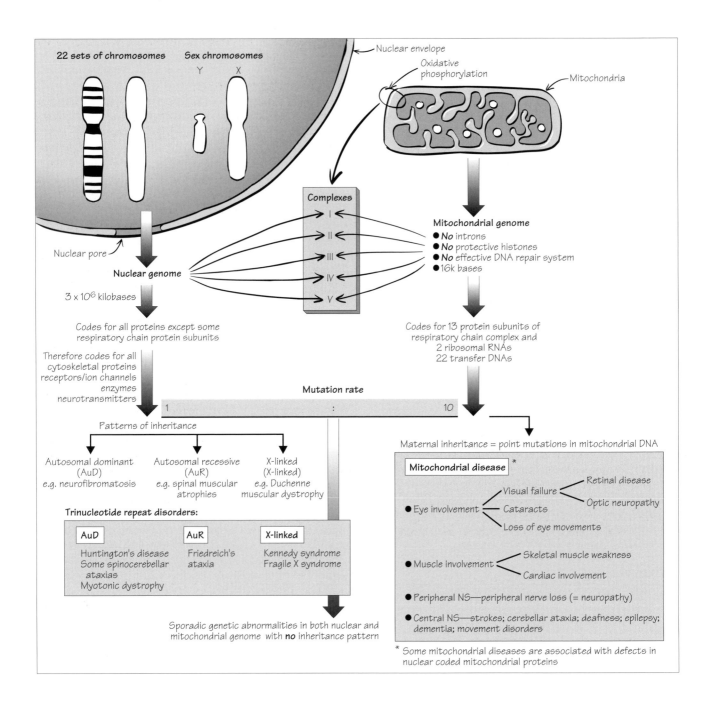

A large number of genetic disorders involve the nervous system, and some of these have pathology confined solely to this structure. Recent advances in molecular genetics have meant that many diseases of the nervous system are being redefined by their underlying genetic defect.

Two major new developments have revolutionized the role of genetic factors in the evolution of neurological disease. First, genes encoded in the maternally inherited **mitochondrial genome** can cause neurological disorders and, secondly, a number of inherited neurological disorders have as their basis an expanded trinucleotide repeat (**triplet repeat disorders**).

Disorders with gene deletions

Many different disorders within the nervous system result from the loss of a single gene or part thereof. For example, *hereditary neuropathy with a liability to pressure palsies*, in which the patient has a tendency to develop recurrent focal entrapment neuropathies in association with a large deletion on chromosome 17, which includes the gene coding for the peripheral myelin protein 22 (PMP 22).

Disorders with gene duplications

The duplication of a gene can, under some circumstances, cause disease. An example of this is in certain types of *hereditary motor and sensory neuropathy*, where the patient develops distal weakness, wasting and sensory loss in the first decades of life. In some of these cases there is duplication of part of chromosome 17, including the gene coding for PMP 22.

Disorders with gene mutations

This is the most common form of genetic defect and in these diseases there is a mutation in the gene coding for a specific enzyme or protein which results in that product failing to work normally.

An example of such a situation is found in some familial forms of *motorneurone disease* (see Chapter 52), *muscular dystrophies* (see Chapter 10) as well as *myotonic syndromes* (see Chapter 5).

Disorders showing genetic imprinting

Genetic imprinting is the differential expression of autosomal genes depending upon their parental origin. Thus, disruption of the maternal gene(s) on a certain part of chromosome 15 (15q11-q13) causes *Prader–Willi syndrome* (mental retardation with obesity, hypogenitalism and short stature) while disruption of the same genes from the father causes *Angelman's syndrome* (a condition of severe mental retardation, cerebellar ataxia, epilepsy and craniofacial abnormalities).

Mitochondrial disorders

Mitochondria contain their own DNA and synthesize a number of the proteins in the respiratory chain responsible for oxidative phosphorylation (see Chapter 52), although the vast majority of mitochondrial proteins are encoded by nuclear DNA. Thus, mitochondrial disorders (deletions, duplication or point mutations) can result from defects in either these nuclear coded genes or the mitochondria genome. However, mitochondrial DNA mutates more than 10 times as frequently as nuclear DNA and has no introns (non-coding parts of the genome), so that a random mutation will usually strike a coding DNA sequence. As mitochondria are inherited from the fertilized oocyte, disorders with point mutations in the mitochondrially coded DNA show maternal inheritance (always inherited from the mother). However, within each cell there are many mitochondria and so a given cell can

contain both normal and mutant mitochondrial DNA, a situation known as **heteroplasmy** and it is only when a given threshold is reached that disease results.

The clinical disorders associated with different defects in the mitochondrial genome are legion, and the reason why some areas are targeted in some conditions and not others is not clear.

Trinucleotide repeat disorders

A number of different disorders have now been identified that have as their major genetic defect an expanded triplet repeat, i.e. there is a large and abnormal expansion of three bases in the genome. In normal individuals triplet repeat sequences are not uncommon but once the number of repeats exceeds a certain number the disease will definitely appear.

This pathological triplet (or trinucleotide) repeat either occurs in the coding part of a gene (e.g. *Huntington's disease*; see Chapter 39) or in a non-coding part of the genome (e.g. *Friedreich's ataxia*). The resulting expansion either causes a loss of function (e.g. frataxin in *Friedreich's ataxia*) or a new gain of function in that gene product (e.g. huntingtin in *Huntington's disease*). This latter aspect is of interest as the new protein appears to have a function that is unique to it and which is critical to the evolution of the neurodegenerative process. However, the mechanism by which this protein produces selective neuronal death in specific CNS sites is not known as many of the mutant gene products are widely expressed throughout the brain and body.

The consequence of a large unstable DNA sequence as occurs in these disorders is that the triplet repeat can increase during mitosis and meiosis, resulting in longer triplet repeat sequences (**dynamic mutations**). This means that the most likely time for triplet expansion is during spermatogenesis and subsequent fertilization/embryogenesis, and has two major implications. First, longer repeats tend to occur in the offspring of affected men and, secondly, longer repeats tend to occur in subsequent generations. This results in patients of subsequent generations presenting with earlier onset and more severe forms of the disorder—a phenomenon known as **genetic anticipation** as longer repeat sequences are associated with younger onset and more severe forms of the disease.

Appendix 1: Major neurotransmitter types

Neurotransmitter	Distribution	Receptor types	Associated neurological disorders
Amino acids *Excitatory*			
Glutamate	Widespread throughout CNS	1. Ionotropic: Non-NMDA (AMPA; kainate; quisqualate receptors) NMDA 2. Metabotropic	Epilepsy (Ch 53) Excitotoxic cell death (Ch 52)
Inhibitory			
GABA	Widespread throughout CNS	$GABA_A$ $GABA_B$	Spinal cord motor disorders (Ch 34) Epilepsy (Ch 53) Anxiety (Ch 51)
Glycine	Spinal cord	Glycine	Startle syndromes (Ch 34)
Monoamines*			
Noradrenaline (nor-epinephrine)	Locus ceruleus to whole CNS (Ch 13) Postganglionic sympathetic nervous system (Ch 42)	$\alpha 1; \alpha 2$ $\beta 1; \beta 2$	Depression (Ch 50) Autonomic failure (Ch 42) Pain (Ch 21, 22)
Serotonin (5-hydroxytryptamine)	Raphe nucleus in brainstem to whole CNS (Ch 50)	$5\text{-}HT_1$ (A–F) $5\text{-}HT_2$ (A–C) $5\text{-}HT_3$–$5\text{-}HT_7$	Depression (Ch 50) Anxiety (Ch 51) Migraine Pain (Ch 21, 22)
Dopamine	Nigrostriatal pathway in basal ganglia (Ch 38) Mesolimbic and mesocortical pathways (Ch 50) Retina (Ch 23) Hypothalamic–pituitary projection (Ch 43)	D1–D5 receptors on activation cause an increase in intracellular cAMP D2 receptors cause a decrease in intracellular cAMP on activation D3–D4 are independent of cAMP signalling system	Parkinson's disease (Ch 39) Schizophrenia (Ch 50) Control of pituitary hormone secretion (Ch 43) Control of vomiting
Acetylcholine	Neuromuscular junction (Ch 7) Autonomic nervous system (Ch 42) Basal forebrain to cerebral cortex and limbic system (Ch 45, 52) Interneurones in many CNS structures including striatum (Ch 38)	Nicotinic Muscarinic (M1–M3 subtypes)	Disorders of the neuromuscular junction (Ch 7) Autonomic failure (Ch 42) Dementia of the Alzheimer type (Ch 52) Parkinson's disease (Ch 39) Epilepsy (Ch 53) Sleep–wake cycle (Ch 44)
Neuropeptides	Widespread distribution in CNS but especially are found in: dorsal horn of spinal cord (Ch 21, 22) basal ganglia (Ch 38) autonomic nervous system (Ch 42)	Various	See: Pain systems (Ch 21, 22) Basal ganglia (Ch 38) Autonomic nervous system (Ch 42) Neural plasticity (Ch 47) Anxiety (Ch 51) Sleep (Ch 44)
Others Purinergic ATP Endozapines			

*Histamine and adrenaline (noradrenaline) are monoamines that are found primarily in the hypothalamus and adrenal medulla respectively.

Appendix 2a: Ascending sensory pathways in spinal cord

Tract	Spinothalamic tract (STT)	Dorsal column–medial lemniscal pathway	Spinocerebellar tract (SCT)
Relevant chapter	21	20	37
Site of origin	Dorsal horn (Laminae I, III, IV and V) Crosses midline in spinal cord	Primary afferents from mechanoreceptors, muscle and joint receptors	Spinal cord interneurones and proprioceptive information from muscle and joint
Termination	Somatotopic organization with more caudal fibres added laterally Projects to brainstem and contralateral thalamus	Somatotopic organization with fibres terminating in dorsal column nuclei of medulla Decussate at this level to form medial lemniscus that synapses in ventroposterior nucleus of the thalamus	Two tracts: Dorsal SCT relays information from muscle and joint receptors via inferior cerebellar peduncle to cerebellum Ventral SCT relays information from spinal cord interneurons via superior cerebellar peduncle to cerebellum
Function	Conveys pain and temperature	Conveys proprioception, light touch and vibration	Conveys proprioceptive information as well as information of on-going activity in spinal cord interneurones

Appendix 2b: Descending motor tracts

Tract	Corticospinal or pyramidal tract (CoST)	Rubrospinal tract (RuST)	Vestibulospinal tract (VeST)	Reticulospinal tract (ReST)
Relevant chapters	32, 34–36	32, 34, 37	32, 34, 37	32, 34, 37
Site of origin	Primary motor cortex (40%) Premotor cortex (30%) Somatosensory cortex (30%)	Magnocellular part of red nucleus in midbrain	Deiter's nucleus in the medulla (part of the vestibular nuclear complex)	Caudal reticular formation in pons and medulla
Major actions	Important in independent fractionated finger movements A role in sensory processing (see Ch 20)	Projects to a similar population of MNs as CoST, namely those concerned with distal motor control Experimentally lesions of this tract produce little deficit unless combined with lesions of the CoST Its existence and significance in humans is debated	Innervates predominantly the extensor and axial muscles, and as such is important in the control of posture and balance	The ReST has both an excitatory and inhibitory input to the spinal cord interneurones and to a lesser extent MNs This pathway is important in damping down activity within the spinal cord such that a loss of this pathway produces profound extensor tone

The tectospinal tract is a relatively minor tract originating from the tectum in the midbrain. It is briefly discussed in Chapter 34.

Appendix 3: Functional and anatomical systems of the cerebellum

System	SpinoCBM or paleoCBM: vermal region ■	SpinoCBM or paleoCBM: paravermal or intermediate region ▨	PontoCBM or neoCBM ☐	VestibuloCBM or ArcheoCBM ■
Major afferent connections	Vestibular nucleus Proximal limb Ia/Ib afferents and interneuronal activity relayed via DSCT and VSCT respectively Visual and auditory information to posterior lobe only	Ia/Ib afferents from distal limb via DSCT Interneuronal activity from distal spinal motor pools relayed in VSCT Primary motor and somatosensory cortex	Posterior parietal cortex Primary and premotor motor cortical area *Both* relayed via pontine nuclei	Semicircular canals via vestibular nucleus Visual information from superior colliculus, lateral geniculate nucleus and primary visual cortex relayed via pontine nuclei
Associated deep cerebellar nucleus	Fastigial	Interpositus (globose and emboliform)	Dentate	—
Major efferent projections	Reticular formation → ReST Vestibular nucleus → VeST (ventromedial descending motor pathways)	Red nucleus (magnocellular part) → RuST VA–VL nucleus of the thalamus → PMC (Brodmann's area 6) and MsI (Brodmann's area 4) → corticospinal tract (Dorsolateral descending motor pathways)	VA–VL nucleus of thalamus → Area 4 and 6 → corticospinal tract Red nucleus (parvocellular part) → inferior olive → CBM (Mollaret's triangle)	Vestibular nucleus → VeST Vestibular nucleus → oculomotor nuclei
Specific role	Control of axial musculature Regulate muscle tone	Distal limb coordination Regulate muscle tone	Motor planning Visual control of movement Minor role in distal limb coordination	Posture Eye movement control

Index

Page numbers in *italics* refer to figures; those in **bold** to tables.

abducens nerve (sixth cranial nerve) *36*, 37
  assessment *104*, 105
acalculia 69
accessory nerve *see* spinal accessory nerve
acetylcholine (ACh) 27, **120**
  in neuromuscular transmission *22*, *23*, 28
  in parasympathetic nervous system 93
acetylcholine receptor (AChR) *22*, *23*
  nicotinic 30
acoustic neuroma 37
actin
  filaments *28*, *29*
  in muscle contraction *30*, *31*
  presynaptic network *22*, *23*
action potential
  generation *20*, *21*
  muscle contraction *30*–1
  neuromuscular/synaptic transmission *22*–3
  propagation *24*–5
acute disseminated encephalomyelitis 117
adaptation *44*, 45
Aδ fibres *50*, *51*
adenosine triphosphate (ATP), hydrolysis *30*, 31
adhalin *28*, *29*
adrenaline **120**
adrenocorticotrophic hormone (ACTH) 95
affective disorders 108–9
afferent fibres (axons) *44*, 45
  entry into spinal cord *32*–3
  Ia *74*, *75*
  Ib *74*, *75*
  II *74*, *75*
afferents
  flexor reflex *76*, 77
  primary 44–5
afferent sensory nerve *44*, 45
agraphia 69
akinetic mutism 99
alar plate *12*, *13*
alcoholism, chronic 95
alexia 69
alien limb 69
allodynia 51
all or nothing phenomenon 21
α EEG activity 96
Alzheimer's disease *see under* dementia
amacrine cells *54*, 55
amine uptake inhibitors 109
amino acids
  excitatory 27, **120**
  inhibitory 27, **120**
ampullae *64*, 65
amygdala *98*, 99
β-amyloid protein 113
amyotrophic lateral sclerosis (ALS) 91, *112*
analgesia *52*, 53
anarthria 63
anencephaly 12, 13
Angelman's syndrome 119
angiography 107
anosmia 67
anterior cerebral arteries (ACAs) *42*, 43
anterior choroidal artery *42*, 43

anterior cingulate cortex *50*, 51, *52*, 78
anterior communicating artery *42*, 43
anterior inferior cerebellar artery (AICA) *42*, 43
anterior (ventral) root *10*, 11, 32
anterior spinal artery *42*, 43
  syndrome *70*, 71
anticipation, genetic 119
antidepressants 109
  in anxiety 110
  in pain management *52*, 53
antidiuretic hormone (ADH) 94
antiepileptic drugs *114*, 115
antigen presenting cells 117
antimuscarinic drugs, in Parkinson's disease 87
antiparkinsonian drugs 86–7
antipsychotics 109
anxiety 110–11
  disorders 110, 111
anxiolytic drugs 110, 111
aphagia 95
aphasia 63
  conduction 63
  see also dysphasia
apoptosis *112*, 113
aqueduct of Sylvius *see* central aqueduct of Sylvius
arachnoid granulations 40
arachnoid mater (membrane) *10*, 11, 40
arcuate fasciculus *62*, 63
ascending reticular activating system 96
association cortices (areas) 45, 68–9
astereognosis 69, 71
astigmatism 55
astrocytes *16*, 17
  axonal growth inhibition 103
  foot processes *16*, 41
astrocytomas 17
asynergy 83
ataxia 83
athetosis 87
attention 105
auditory cortex
  primary (A1) *62*, 63
  secondary areas *62*, 63
auditory pathways 62–3
auditory system 60–3
auditory transduction *46*, 47
autoimmune disorders *112*, 113
autonomic failure, pure 93
autonomic nervous system (ANS) 11, 92–3
  anatomy *92*, 93
  CNS control *92*, 93
  damage 93
  hypothalamic control *92*, 93, 94–5
axolemma *14*, 15
axon collaterals *14*, 15
axon hillock *14*, 15
axons *14*, 15
  initial segment *14*, 15
  myelinated *24*, 25
  regeneration *100*, 101
  unmyelinated *24*–5
  Wallerian degeneration *100*, 101

axoplasm *14*, 15
axoplasmic flow (axonal transport) 15

ballismus 73, 87
basal ganglia *10*, 11, 84–5
  diseases 86–7, *90*, 91
  eye movement control 89
  loops 84
  motor control 72–3
  neurophysiology 85
  nociceptive function *50*, 51, *52*
  ventral extension 85
basal plate *12*, 13
basilar artery *42*, 43
basilar membrane (BM) *60*, 61
basket cells, cerebellar (BaC) *82*
Becker's muscular dystrophy 29
Bell's palsy 37
benzodiazepines 97
  in anxiety 110, 111
  dependence/withdrawal syndrome 111
berry aneurysms 43
β-adrenoceptor antagonists (β-blockers) 110, 111
β EEG activity 96
Betz cells *78*, *80*
biopsy
  brain 107
  nerve/muscle 107
bipolar cells *54*, 55
  centre surround receptive field *54*, 55
  off- and on-centre 55
bipolar disorder 108
bitemporal hemianopia *56*, 57
bitter taste *66*, 67
blindsight 59
blind spot *54*, 55
blobs, visual cortex *58*, 59
blood–brain barrier (BBB) *16*, 17, 41, 116
blood supply, CNS *42*, 43
blood tests *106*
bone morphogenic proteins (BMPs) *12*, 13
botulinum toxin *22*, 23
bradykinesia 86
brain
  biopsy 107
  blood supply *42*, 43
  development *12*, 13
  lesions
    motor disorders *90*, 91
    sensory disturbances *70*, 71
  venous drainage 43
brain derived neurotrophic factor (BDNF) *100*
brainstem *10*, 11
  anatomy *34*, 35
  cranial nerves *34*, 35, *36*
  development *12*, 13
  lesions 35, 71
Broca's area *42*, *62*, 63
Brodmann's cytoarchitectural map 38
Brown–Séquard syndrome *70*, 71
bulbar palsy 37

Ca²⁺
  in muscle contraction   30, 31
  in sensory transduction   *46*, 47
  in synaptic transmission   22–3
Ca²⁺ channels, voltage-dependent   22
caloric testing   65
capsaicin   53
carbamazepine   115
carpal tunnel syndrome   71
cataplexy   97
cataracts   55
catecholamine-*O*-methyl-transferase (COMT)
      inhibitors   87
cauda equina   32
caudate nucleus   84
cell death, mechanisms   *112*, 113
cell membrane
  ion channels   18–19
  neuronal   15
central aqueduct of Sylvius   *34, 35, 40*
central aqueduct stenosis   41
central motor conduction time (CMCT)   107
central nervous system (CNS)   *10*, 11
  blood supply   *42*, 43
  control of autonomic nervous system   92, 93
  disorders of embryogenesis   13
  immunological disorders   117
  immunological network   116–17
  plasticity   100, 102–3
  regenerative capacity   103
central pattern generators (CPGs)   73, 76, 77
centre surround receptive field   *54, 55, 58, 59*
cerebellar peduncles   *34, 35*
cerebellum (CBM)   *10*, 11, 82–3
  damage   83, 91
  development   13
  eye movements and   89
  function   83
  motor control   *72, 73*
  organization   *82, 83*, **122**
cerebral cortex   *10*, 11, 38–9
  anatomical organization   38–9
  association areas   45, 68–9
  development   13
  developmental organization   39
  functional organization   39
  motor areas   78–9
  neurophysiological organization   39
  sensory areas   45
cerebral haemorrhage   43
cerebral hemispheres   *10*, 11
cerebral palsy, choreoathetoid   87
cerebral peduncles   *34, 35*
cerebrospinal fluid (CSF)   40–1
  analysis   *106*, 107
  disorders   41
  production and circulation   40–1
cerebrovascular accident (CVA)   63, 81, 91
cervical nerves   *10*, 11
C fibres   *50, 51*
chain fibres   *74, 75*
chemotransduction   *46*, 47
cholecystokinin (CCK₄)   110, 111
chorda tympani   37, 67
chorea   73, 87, 91
choroid plexus   40
  papillomas   17
ciliary ganglion   *56*
cingulate gyrus   98, 99
circadian rhythms   95
circle of Willis   *42, 43*

cisterna magna   40
cisterns, subarachnoid   40
cleft substance   *22*
climbing fibres (cf)   *82, 83, 102*, 103
clonazepam   115
clonus   77
clozapine   109
CNS *see* central nervous system
cochlea   60–1
cochlear nucleus   *62, 63*
codeine   53
cognitive examination   104–5
cognitive impairment *see* dementia
colour blindness   55
columns, cortical   38, 39
  primary auditory cortex   63
  primary motor cortex   81
  primary visual cortex   *58, 59*
common peroneal nerve entrapment   71
complex cells, visual cortex   *58, 59*
computerized tomography (CT)   107
concentration   105
conductance, ion   19
cones   *54, 55*
confabulation   95
coordination *see under* movements
cortical dysplasia   13
cortical plate   39
corticobulbar tracts   78
corticospinal tract (CoST, pyramidal tract)   49,
      121
  cortical projections   78
  damage   77
  in motor control   *72, 73, 76, 77*
  spinal cord   *32, 33*
corticotrophin-releasing hormone (CRH)   111
cotransmission   25
cranial nerves   11, 36–7
  brainstem components   *34, 35, 36*
  examination   *104*, 105
  see also specific nerves
Creutzfeldt–Jakob disease   113
cribriform plate   *66, 67*
critical firing threshold   *20, 21*
critical period (of development)   102–3
crossbridges, actin–myosin   30, 31
cuneate nucleus   *48, 49*
curare   *22, 23*
current, ion   19
cyclic adenosine monophosphate (cAMP)   *46,
      47*
cyclic guanosine monophosphate (cGMP)   *46,
      47*

deafness
  conductive   *60, 61*
  congenital   47
  sensorineural   *60, 61*
decerebrate posture   77
decibels (dB)   *60, 61*
decussation, ascending sensory pathways   33
deep-brain stimulation, for Parkinson's disease
      87
deep cerebellar nuclei neurones (DCCN)   *82, 83*
dementia
  of Alzheimer type (DAT)   27, 99, *112*, 113
  in basal ganglia disorders   87
  frontotemporal   *112*
demyelinating neuropathies   17, 117
dendrites   *14, 15*
dendritic spines   *14, 15*

dentate gyrus   98
depolarization   *20, 21*
depression   108–9
dermatomyositis   117
descending motor pathways *see* motor pathways,
      descending
desensitization, receptor   27
dextropropoxyphene   53
diabetes insipidus   94
diazepam   110, 111
diencephalon   *12, 13*
diplopia   36, 37, 89
distributed system theory   39
dopa decarboxylase inhibitors   86
dopamine (DA)   **120**
  neurone   *108*
  pathways   *108*
    abnormalities in schizophrenia   *108*, 109
  replacement therapy   86–7
dopamine agonists   87
dopamine antagonists   109
dopaminergic nigrostriatal tract   84, 86
dorsal acoustic striae   *62, 63*
dorsal column–medial lemniscal pathway   *48,
      49*, **121**
dorsal column nuclei (DCN)   *34, 35, 48, 49*
dorsal columns   *32, 33*, 49
  electrical stimulation   *52, 53*
dorsal horn   32–3, 49
  nociceptive pathways   *50, 51*
  pain pharmacology   *52, 53*
  sensory processing   33
dorsal root   *10, 11*, 32
dorsal root ganglia (DRG)   *10, 11, 12*
  lesions   71
dorsal spinocerebellar tract (DSCT)   *76, 77*
down-regulation, receptor   27
Duchenne's muscular dystrophy (DMD)   29
dura mater   *10, 11, 40*
dysarthria   63, 83
  scanning   83
dysdiadochokinesis   83
dysmetria   83
dysphasia
  conductive   62
  expressive or non-fluent   *62, 63*
  receptive or fluent   *62, 63*
dyspraxia   43, 105
dystonia   23, 73, 87, 91
dystrophin   28, 29

ear   60–1
  external   *60, 61*
  inner   *60, 61*
  middle   *60, 61*
eardrum   *60, 61*
Edinger–Westphal nucleus   *56, 57*
EE cells, superior olivary complex   *62, 63*
EI cells, superior olivary complex   *62, 63*
eighth cranial nerve *see* vestibulocochlear nerve
electrical tests   107
electrocardiography (ECG)   107
electroencephalography (EEG)   107
  in epilepsy   114
  sleep patterns   96
electromyography (EMG)   107
eleventh cranial nerve *see* spinal accessory nerve
embryogenesis
  disorders of CNS   13
  nervous system   12–13
encephalitis   *116*

encephalomyelitis
   acute disseminated 117
   experimental allergic 117
endocytosis, synaptic vesicles 23
endolymph *64*, 65
endoneurial tubes 101
endorphins 51
endothelial cells, blood–brain barrier *16*, 41
end-plate potential (epp) *22*, 23
end-stopped cells, visual cortex *58*, 59
enkephalins 51
entacapone 87
enteric nervous system 93
entorhinal cortex 98
ependymal cells *16*, 17
ependymomas 17
epilepsy 27, 114–15
   Jacksonian 81, 91
   pathogenesis 19, 114–15
   primary generalized *114*, 115
   sensory features 45
   temporal lobe 67, 99, *114*, 115
   treatment *114*, 115
equilibrium potential *20*, 21
ethosuximide 115
evoked potentials (EPs) 107
examination, nervous system 104–5
excitatory amino acids 27, **120**
excitatory postsynaptic potentials (EPSPs) 25
excitatory synapses *24*, 25
excitotoxic cell death *112*, 113
experimental allergic encephalomyelitis 117
external auditory meatus *60*, 61
external cerebral veins 43
extinction 69
extraocular muscles *88*
extrapyramidal tracts 33, *72*, 73
eye 54–5
   optical properties 54–5
   reverse suturing 103
eye movements 88–9
   in basal ganglia lesions 87
   CNS control 89
   reflex 89
   saccadic 57, 89
   types 89
   voluntary 89

facial nerve (seventh cranial nerve) *36*, 37
   assessment *104*, 105
   palsy 37
F-actin *28*, 29
feature detection 45
feedback inhibition *24*, 25
feeding, control of 95
fetal nigral transplants, for Parkinson's disease 87
fifth cranial nerve *see* trigeminal nerve
first cranial nerve *see* olfactory nerve
flexor reflex afferents *76*, 77
foot drop *70*, 71
foramen magnum 11
foramen of Munro *40*
foramina of Luschka and Magendie *40*
fourth cranial nerve *see* trochlear nerve
fourth ventricle *40*
fovea *54*, 55
free radicals *112*, 113
frequency coding 45
Friedreich's ataxia 119
frontal eye fields (FEF)

eye movements and 89
   in motor control 78, 79
frontal lobe *10*, 11
   function, assessment 104–5
   lesions 69
   in motor control 78–9
functional magnetic resonance imaging (fMRI) 107

GABA *see* γ-aminobutyric acid
GABA$_A$ receptors 97
gabapentin 115
gag reflex 105
gait disorders 77
γ-aminobutyric acid (GABA) 27, **120**
   in anxiety 110
   in epileptic seizures 114, 115
γ-aminobutyric acid
   (GABA)–benzodiazepine–barbiturate
   receptor 26
ganglion *10*, 11
ganglion cells, retinal *54*, 55
   lateral geniculate nucleus projections *56*, 57
   XYW system 55
gap junctions 23
gate theory of pain 53
gaze, sustained 89
gemmules *14*, 15
gene
   deletions 118
   duplications 118–19
   mutations 119
generalized anxiety disorder 110, 111
genetic disorders 118–19
glial cell line derived neurotrophic factor
   (GDNF) 101, 113
glial cells *16*, 17
   see also astrocytes; microglial cells;
      oligodendrocytes
glia limitans 17
globus pallidus
   external (GPe) 84
   internal (GPi) 84
glossopharyngeal (ninth) nerve *36*, 37, 67
   assessment *104*, 105
'glove and stocking' pattern of sensory loss 71
glutamate 27, **120**
glutamate receptors 27
   ionotropic 27
   in long-term potentiation *98*, 99
   metabotropic 27
glutamic acid decarboxylase (GAD) antibodies 77
glycine 27, **120**
Golgi cells, cerebellar (GoC) *82*, 83
Golgi tendon organ 73, *74*, 75
G protein, olfactory receptor-associated (G$_{olf}$) *46*, 47
gracile nucleus *48*, 49
'grandmother' cells 39
granule cells, cerebellar (GrC) *82*, 83
grey matter *10*, 11
growth cone 12
Guillain–Barré syndrome 19, 25, 93, *116*, 117
gustatory receptors *66*, 67
gustatory transduction *66*, 67
gustducin *66*, 67

hair cells
   cochlea *46*, 47, *60*, 61

otolith *64*, 65
   semicircular canal *64*, 65
heavy meromyosin (HMM) *28*, 29
helicotrema *60*, 61
hemianopia
   bitemporal *56*, 57
   homonymous *56*, 57
hemiballismus 87, 91
hemiparesis 77, 91
hemiplegia 77
hereditary motor sensory neuropathy (HMSN) 23, 119
hereditary neuropathy with a liability to pressure
   palsies 118
heteroplasmy 119
hierarchy
   cortical cell organization 39
   motor system 72–3
high-threshold mechanoreceptors (HTM) 51
hippocampal complex *98*, 99
hippocampus *10*, 11, *98*, 99
   CA1–CA4 subfields *98*, 99
   neural progenitor cells 13
histamine **120**
history taking 106
HIV infection 113
horizontal cells *54*, 55
Horner's syndrome 93
Huntington's disease *86*, 87, 113, 119
hydrocephalus 17, 41, 91
   compensatory 41
   obstructive 41
5-hydroxytryptamine (5-HT) *see* serotonin
hyperalgesia
   primary 51
   secondary 51
hypercolumns, visual cortex *58*, 59
hypercomplex cells, visual cortex *58*, 59
hyperekplexia 27
hypermetropia 54–5
hyperphagia 95
hyperpolarization *20*, 21
hyperreflexia 77
hypersomnia 97
hyperthermia/hyperpyrexia, malignant 31
hypertonia 77
hypnotic drugs 97
hypocretins *96*, 97
hypoglossal (twelfth) nerve *36*, 37
   assessment *104*, 105
hypotension
   orthostatic 93
   postprandial 93
hypothalamus 51, 94–5
   autonomic control *92*, 93, 94–5
   control of sleep *96*, 97
   functions 94–5
   olfactory projections *66*, 67
   suprachiasmatic nucleus 57, 95
hypotonia 83

imaging 106–7
immunological disorders 116–17
immunological privilege 116
imprinting, genetic 119
inattention (neglect) 69, 71
incoordination 83, 91
infections
   causing neurodegeneration *112*, 113
   intrauterine 13
inferior colliculus (IC) *34*, 35, *62*, 63

inferior olive *34*, 35
inflammatory disorders 116–17
inheritance, patterns *118*
inhibitory amino acids 27, **120**
inhibitory Ia interneurones (INs) *74*, 75, 77
inhibitory postsynaptic potentials (IPSPs) *24*, 25
inhibitory synapses *24*, 25
inner hair cells (IHC) *60*, 61
input–output coupling, primary motor cortex 81
insomnia 97
insular cortex *50*, 51, *52*
interblobs, visual cortex *58*, 59
interictal activity 114
intermanual conflict 69
internal carotid arteries (ICAs) *42*, 43
internal cerebral veins 43
interneurones (IN)
  Ia inhibitory *74*, 75, 77
  spinal cord 73, 76
internuclear ophthalmoplegia 89
intracerebral haemorrhage 43
intracranial pressure, raised 41
investigations, nervous system 106–7
ion channels 18–19
  chemically activated (ligand gated) 18, 19
  clinical disorders 19
  modulation *18*, 19
  receptors coupled to *18*, 19, 26
  selectivity filter *18*, 19
  voltage gated 18, 19
Isaac's syndrome (neuromyotonia) 22, 23

Jacksonian march (epilepsy) 81, 91
joint position sense (JPS) (proprioception) 75
  testing *104*, 105

K⁺, resting membrane potential and *20*, 21
K⁺ channels, voltage gated *20*, 21
keratitis 55
Korsakoff's syndrome 95

labyrinth *64*, 65
labyrinthitis 65
lacunar infarcts 43
Lambert–Eaton myasthenic syndrome 22, 23, *116*, 117
laminae of Rexed 32
laminar organization, cerebral cortex 38–9
lamotrigine 115
language 62–3
  assessment 105
lateral geniculate nucleus (LGN) 56, 57, 58–9
lateral inhibition 33, *44*, 45
lateral medullary syndrome of Wallenberg 43
lateral motor system *76*, 77
lateral popliteal nerve entrapment 71
lateral ventricles *40*
levodopa (L-dopa) 86–7
Lewy bodies 86
light meromyosin (LMM) *28*, 29
limb girdle muscular dystrophies (LGMD) 29
limbic system 98–9
  motor control 72
  olfactory projections *66*, 67
limbs, motor examination *104*, 105
local anaesthetics, in pain management 53
locomotion 76–7
  disorders 77
  fictive 77
locus ceruleus *50*, 51, *96*, 97

long-latency reflexes 81
long-sightedness 54–5
long-term depression (LTD) 27, 83, 99, 103
long-term potentiation (LTP) 27, 98–9
Lou Gehrig disease (amyotrophic lateral sclerosis) 91, *112*
lower motorneurones (LMNs) 73, 74–5
  lesions 73, 75, *90*, 91
lumbar nerves *10*, 11
lumbar puncture *106*, 107

magnetic resonance angiography/venography (MRA/MRV) 107
magnetic resonance imaging (MRI) 107
  functional 107
magnocellular laminae/cells 56, 57, *58*
major histocompatibility complex (MHC) antigens 116–17
malignant hyperthermia/hyperpyrexia 31
mammillary bodies 95, 98
mania 108
M channels 57, *58*, 59
mechanoelectrical transduction *46*, 47
mechanoreceptors, high-threshold (HTM) 51
medial geniculate nucleus (MGN) *62*, 63
medial lemniscus *34*, 35, *48*, 49
medial longitudinal fasciculus (MLF) *34*, 35, 89
  rostral interstitial nucleus (riMLF) 89
median nerve entrapment 71
medulla *10*, 11, *34*, 35
Meissner's corpuscles *48*, 49
memory 95, 98–9
  anterograde 105
meninges *10*, 11, 40–1
meningiomas 41, 67
meningism 41
meningitis 41, *116*
  malignant 41
meningocoele 13
meningomyelocoele 13
Merkel's discs *48*, 49
meromyosin proteins *28*, 29
mesencephalon *12*, 13
metabolic myopathies 31
metencephalon *12*, 13
microfilaments 15
microglial cells 17, 117
microtubules 15
midbrain *10*, 11, *34*, 35
middle cerebral arteries (MCAs) *42*, 43
migraine 45
  familial hemiplegic 19
miniature end-plate potential (mepp) 22, 23
mitochondria
  genome 118
  neuronal *14*, 15
mitochondrial disorders 87, *118*, 119
moclobemide 109
Mollaret triangle damage 83
monoamine neurotransmitters 27, **120**
monoamine oxidase inhibitors (MAOIs) 109
monoamine theory of depression 109
monocular deprivation *102*, 103
morphine 53
mossy fibres *82*, 83, *98*, 99
motor cortex, primary (MsI) 78, **79**, 80–1
  lesions **79**, 81
  organization 81
motor cortical areas 78–9
motor homunculus 78, *80*, 81

motorneurone disease (MND) 63, 91, 101, *112*, 113
motorneurones (MNs) 73
  α 33, 74–5
    damage to 75, 101
  γ 33, *74*, 75
  lateral pool *76*, 77
  recruitment 75
  spinal 32, 33, *76*, 77
  upper (UMN), lesions 73, *90*, 91
  ventromedial pool *76*, 77
  see also lower motorneurones
motor pathways, descending 73, 76–7, **121**
  lesions 77, 91
  spinal cord tracts *32*, 33
motor system 72–3
  basal ganglia function 84, 85
  cerebellar function 83
  cortical areas 78–81
  disorders 90–1
  examination *104*, 105
  hierarchy 72–3
  lateral *76*, 77
  spinal *see* spinal cord, motor control
  ventromedial *76*, 77
motor unit 74
movements
  closed-loop (reflexly controlled) 72
  coding for direction and force 81
  coordination 73, 83
    assessment 105
  disorders 73, 83, 90–1
  initiation, planning and programming 72–3
  open-loop (volitional) 72
multiple sclerosis 17, 19, 117
  cerebellar damage 91
  eye movement disorders 89
  nerve conduction abnormalities 25
  trigeminal neuralgia 53
  vestibular dysfunction 65
multiple-system atrophy 93
muscle
  antagonist *74*, 75
  biopsy 107
  contraction 30–1
  disorders 29, 31, 90–1
  homonymous *74*, 75
  inflammatory disorders *116*, 117
  power *104*, 105
  structure 28–9
  synergistic *74*, 75
  tone *104*, 105
muscle fibres 28–9
  extrafusal *74*, 75
  intrafusal *74*, 75
muscle spindle 73, 74–5
  damage to afferent fibres 75
muscular dystrophies 29, 90–1
mutations 119
  dynamic 119
mutism, akinetic 99
myalgia 90
myasthenia gravis 22, 23, 91, *116*, 117
myelencephalon *12*, 13
myelin
  nerve conduction and 24, 25
  sheath *14*, 15
myelinated axons (fibres) *24*, 25
myelitis *116*
  transverse *70*, 71
myelography 107

myoclonus, palatal 83
myofibrils 28
myopia 54–5
myosin 28–9, 30
myositis *116*
myotonia 19

Na$^+$, resting membrane potential and *20*, 21
Na$^+$ channels, voltage gated *18*, *20*, 21
Na$^+$–K$^+$ exchange pump *20*, 21
naloxone 53
narcolepsy 97
neglect (inattention) 69, 71
neocortex *see* cerebral cortex
neostriatum (NS) *84*, 85
Nernst equation *20*, 21
nerve biopsy 107
nerve conduction 24–5
    block 25
    disorders of 25
    studies (NCS) *106*, 107
nerve entrapments, focal *70*, 71
nerve fibres *see* axons
nerve growth factor (NGF) *100*, 101
nerve impulse *see* action potential
nerve root (radicular) syndromes *70*, 71
nerve terminal *14*, 15
nervous system
    cells 14–17
    development 12–13
    examination 104–5
    investigation 106–7
    organization *10*, 11
neural crest 12
neural groove 12
neural plate 12
neural stem (progenitor) cells 13, 103
neural tube 12–13
neuritis *116*
neuroblasts 13
neurochemical disorders 108–11
neurodegenerative disorders 112–13
neurofibrillary tangles (NFTs) 113
neurofibromatosis type I 17
neurofilaments *14*, 15
neurogenesis, adult 13
neurogenetic disorders 118–19
neuroglial cells *16*, 17
neuroimmunological disorders 116–17
neuroleptics 109
neurological examination 104–5
neuroma 51
neuromodulation 26
neuromuscular junction (NMJ) *14*, 22–3
    disorders 22, 23, *90*, 91
    immunological disorders *116*, 117
neuromuscular transmission 28
neuromyotonia 22, 23
neurones 14–15
    cell body (soma) *14*–15
    multipolar 15
    pseudo-unipolar 15
neuropathies *see* peripheral neuropathies
neuropeptides 27, **120**
    in anxiety 111
neuroses 110
neurotoxins *112*, 113
neurotransmitters 26–7, **120**
    diversity and anatomy of pathways 27
    inactivation (hydrolysis or uptake) 23, 26–7
    in synaptic transmission 22, 23, 25

neurotrophic factors 100–3
    in neurodegenerative disorders *112*,
        113
neurotrophins *100*, 101
night blindness 47
nigrostriatal tract, dopaminergic 84, 86
ninth cranial nerve *see* glossopharyngeal nerve
Nissl substance. *14*, 15
N-methyl-D-aspartate (NMDA) receptors 27,
    99
nociception 51
nociceptive pathways *50*, 51
nociceptors *50*, 51
    polymodal (PMN) 51
nodes of Ranvier *14*, *15*, 24, 25
noise 45
non-NMDA receptors 27
noradrenaline (norepinephrine) 93, **120**
    abnormalities in depression 109
    in anxiety 111
notochord 12
nuclear bag fibres *74*, 75
nucleus accumbens 85, 96
nucleus ambiguus *34*, 35
nucleus of lateral lemniscus (NLL) *62*, 63
nucleus of solitary tract 67
nucleus raphe interpositus 89
numbness 70
nystagmus 83, 89

obstructive sleep apnoea syndrome 97
occipital lobe *10*, 11
ocular dominance (OD) columns *58*, 59, *102*,
    103
oculomotor nerve (III) 36
    assessment *104*, 105
oculomotor nuclei *88*, 89
odour 67
olfaction 66–7
olfactory bulb *66*, 67
olfactory nerve (I) 36, 67
    assessment 105
olfactory receptors *66*, 67
olfactory tract *66*, 67
olfactory transduction *46*, 47
oligodendrocytes 15, *16*, 17
    axonal growth inhibition 103
oligodendroglioma 17
ophthalmoplegia, internuclear 89
opioid analgesics *52*, 53
opioids, endogenous 51
opsoclonus 89
optic chiasm 56
optic disc 55
optic nerve (II) 36, *56*
    assessment *104*, 105
optic tract 56
optokinetic reflex 89
orexins 97
organ of Corti *60*, 61
orientation in time, person and place 104
orientation selective columns *58*, 59
oscillopsia 65, 89
osmoregulation 95
ossicles, auditory *60*, 61
otitis media 61
otolith organs *64*, 65
otosclerosis 61
outer hair cells (OHC) *60*, 61
oval window *60*, 61
oxytocin 94

Pacinian corpuscles *48*, 49
pain 50–3
    chronic 51, 53
    defined 51
    management 52–3
    pathways *50*, 51
    pharmacology 52–3
    pinprick testing 105
    referred 51
    syndromes 53, 71
    systems 50–1
    transduction 51
palatal tremor/myoclonus 83
pallidotomy, for Parkinson's disease 87
pallidum, ventral 85
panic attacks 111
panic disorder 110
paraesthesiae 70
parahippocampal structures 98, 99
parallel fibres, cerebellar *82*, 83
parallel pathways 39
paramedian pontine reticular formation (PPRF)
    89
paraneoplastic syndromes 101, 113, 117
paraproteinaemias *116*, 117
parasubiculum 98
parasympathetic nervous system *92*, 93
    pupils *56*, 57
parietal cortex, posterior *see* posterior parietal
        cortex
parietal lobe *10*, 11
    function, assessment 105
parkinsonism 87, 113
Parkinson's disease 73, 79, 86–7, 91, *112*
    eye movement abnormalities 89
    pathogenesis 27, 84, 86, 113
    treatment 86–7, 113
parvocellular laminae/cells 56, 57, *58*
pattern generators, central 73, 76, 77
P channels 57, *58*, 59
pedunculopontine nucleus (PPN) 84
peptides *see* neuropeptides
periaqueductal grey matter (PAG) *34*, 35, *50*,
    51
periodic paralyses 19, 31
peripheral nerves 11
    immunological disorders 117
    lesions
        chronic pain syndromes 53, 71
        motor disturbances 91
        sensory disorders *70*, 71
    regeneration 100–1
    sectioning, in pain management *52*, 53
peripheral nervous system (PNS) 11
    plasticity 100–1
peripheral neuropathies 49, 71
    generalized *70*, 71
    large fibre 75
perirhinal cortex 98
permeability, ion channel 19
pernicious anaemia 71
phenobarbital 115
phenytoin 115
phobias 110, 111
photopic vision 55
photopigments *54*, 55
photoreceptors *54*, 55
phototransduction *46*, 47
pia mater *10*, 11, 40
pinprick testing 105
pituitary gland 94

pituitary tumours 94
plantar responses *104*, 105
plasticity
  central nervous system 100, 102–3
  peripheral nervous system 100–1
poliomyelitis 91, 101
polymodal nociceptors (PMN) 51
polymyositis 117
pons *10*, 11, *34*, 35
pore, transmembrane 19
positron emission tomography (PET) 107
posterior cerebral arteries (PCAs) *42*, 43
posterior communicating artery *42*, 43
posterior fossa 11
posterior inferior cerebellar artery (PICA) *42*, 43
posterior parietal cortex (PPC) *48*, 49, 68–9
  area 5 68–9
  area 7 *68*, 69
  eye movement control 89
  lesions 69, *70*, 71
  motor control *72*, 78, 79
posterior root *see* dorsal root
posterior spinal arteries *42*, 43
postherpetic neuralgia 53
postsubiculum 98
postsynaptic membrane *14*, 15, 22
postsynaptic receptors 22, *23*, 25, 26–7
postsynaptic secondary (junctional) folds 22
power, muscle *104*, 105
Prader–Willi syndrome 119
prefrontal cortex *50*, 51, *52*, 68–9
pregnancy, anticonvulsant drugs in 115
premotor cortex (PMC) *72*, 78, 79
  lesions **79**, 81
presubiculum 98
presynaptic active zones 22
presynaptic autoreceptors 25, 26
presynaptic inhibition 25
presynaptic membrane 22, *23*
presynaptic nerve terminal (bouton, end-bulb) *14*, 15, 22
presynaptic vesicles 22, *23*
pretectal nuclei *56*, 57
primary afferents 44–5
primary sensory cortex 45
programmed cell death (apoptosis) *112*, 113
proprioception *see* joint position sense
propriospinal neurones *76*, 77
prosencephalon *12*, 13
pseudobulbar palsy 37
psychiatric disorders 108–11
psychotherapy, supportive 110
ptosis 36
pupillary defect, relative afferent 57
pupillary light response 36, *56*, 57
Purkinje cells, cerebellar (PuC) *82*, 83, *102*, 103
putamen 84
pyramid *34*, 35
pyramidal distribution of weakness 73, 77
pyramidal tract *see* corticospinal tract
pyriform cortex *66*, 67

quadrantanopia *56*, 57

radial glial fibres 13, *39*
radicular syndromes *70*, 71
raphe nuclei *50*, 51, 96–7, 111

rapid eye movement (REM) sleep 96
receptive field 45
  centre surround (circular symmetric) organization *54*, 55, *58*, 59
receptors 26–7
  desensitization and downregulation 27
  ion channel-coupled *18*, 19, 26
  membrane enzyme coupled 26
  postsynaptic *see* postsynaptic receptors
  super-sensitivity and up-regulation 27
recoverin 46
recruitment 45
  motorneurone, principle of 75
recurrent artery of Heubner 43
red nucleus *34*, 35
reflexes
  assessment *104*, 105
  long-latency or transcortical 81
  motor 73
  primitive 105
  stretch 73
  tendon 75, 105
reflex sympathetic dystrophy *52*, 53, 93
refraction *54*–5
refractory period 21
  absolute 21
  relative 21
relative afferent pupillary defect 57
Renshaw cells *76*, 77
resting membrane potential *20*, 21
reticular activating system, ascending 96
reticular formation 96–7
  paramedian pontine (PPRF) 89
reticulospinal tract (ReST) 73, **121**
  in motor control *76*, 77
  spinal cord *32*, 33
retina *54*–5
  anatomy and function *54*, 55
  ascending projections 56–7, *58*–9
  phototransduction *46*, 47
retinitis pigmentosa 55
retinotopic organization 56–7, *58*–9
Rexed's laminae 32
rhodopsin *46*, *54*
rhombencephalon *12*, 13
rigidity, cogwheel 86
risperidone 109
rods *54*, 55
rostral migratory stream (RMS) 13
rubrospinal tract (RuST) 73, **121**
  in motor control *76*, 77
  spinal cord *32*, 33
Ruffini endings *48*, 49
ryanodine receptor abnormalities 31

saccadic eye movements 57, 89
sacculus *64*, 65
sacral nerves *10*, 11
saltatory conduction *24*, 25
salt taste *66*, 67
sarcoglycan complex *28*, 29
sarcolemma 28
sarcomere *28*, 29
sarcoplasmic reticulum (SR) *28*, 31
satiety centre 95
scala media *60*, 61
scala tympani *60*, 61
scala vestibuli *60*, 61
Scarpa's ganglion *64*, 65
schizophrenia 108–9

Schwann cells 15, *16*, 17
  in peripheral nerve repair *100*, 101
schwannomas 17
scotopic vision 55
secondary sensory areas 45
second cranial nerve *see* optic nerve
seizures *114*
  complex partial 114
  generalized 114
  partial 114
  see also epilepsy
selective serotonin reuptake inhibitors (SSRIs) 109
selegiline 87
semicircular canals *64*, 65
senile neuritic plaques (SNPs) 113
sensory afferent fibres *see* afferent fibres
sensory cortical areas, primary and secondary 45
sensory examination *104*, 105
sensory homunculus 49
sensory pathways 45
  clinical disorders 45, 70–1
  spinal cord *32*, 33, **121**
sensory receptors 44–5
  cutaneous *48*, 49
  sensitivity 45
  threshold 45
sensory symptoms 70
sensory systems 44–5
  specificity or modality 45
sensory transduction 44, 46–7
septal nuclei 98
serotonin (5-HT) **120**
  abnormalities in depression 109
  neurones *108*
  pathways *108*, 111
  role in anxiety 110, 111
seventh cranial nerve *see* facial nerve
short-sightedness *54*–5
signal to noise ratio 45
simple cells, visual cortex *58*, 59
single positron emission tomography (SPECT) 107
sixth cranial nerve *see* abducens nerve
size principle 75
skin, sensory receptors *48*, 49
sleep 96–7
  disorders 97
  neural mechanisms 96–7
  non-rapid eye movement (non-REM) 96
  rapid eye movement (REM) 96
  slow-wave (SWS) 96
sleep apnoea, obstructive 97
sleepiness, daytime 97
sliding filament hypothesis, muscle contraction 30, 31
smooth pursuit eye movements 89
somatosensory cortex
  primary (SmI) *48*, 49, 51
    lesions *70*, 71
  secondary (SmII) *48*, 49, 51
somatosensory system 44, 45, 48–9
  disorders 49
  plasticity 103
somatotopic organization 33
sonic hedgehog *12*, 13
sound
  amplitude (loudness) *60*, 61

frequency (pitch) *60*, 61
frequency tuning *62*, 63
localization *62*, 63
transduction *46*, 47
waves, properties *60*, 61
sour taste *66*, 67
spatial coding 45
spatial summation *24*, 25
spina bifida 12, 13
hydrocephalus 41
occulta 13
spinal accessory (eleventh) nerve *36*, 37
assessment *104*, 105
spinal cord *10*, 11, 32–3
ascending (sensory) pathways *32*, 33, **121**
blood supply *42*, 43
descending pathways *see* motor pathways, descending
development 12–13
dorsal columns *see* dorsal columns
dorsal horn *see* dorsal horn
intermediate zone (lateral column) *10*, 11, 32
lesions 33
motor syndromes 77, *90*, 91
sensory syndromes *70*, 71
motor control *72*, 73
disorders 77, *90*, 91
organization 76–7
nociceptive pathways *50*, 51
subacute combined degeneration *70*, 71
ventral horn *32*, 33
spinal nerves 11
spinocerebellar tract *32*, 33, **121**
dorsal (DSCT) *76*, 77
ventral (VSCT) *76*, 77
spinomesencephalic tract 51
spinoreticulothalamic tract *50*, 51
spinothalamic tract (STT) *50*, 51, **121**
lesions *70*, 71
spinal cord *32*, 33
stance phase, locomotion *76*, 77
stearic block 29, 30
stellate cells, cerebellar (StC) *82*
stem cells, neural 13, 103
step 77
stereocilia
in auditory transduction *46*, 47
in vestibular transduction *64*, 65
stiff-person syndrome 77, 91
stress reactions 110
stretch reflex 73
striatum
dorsal (neostriatum, NS) *84*, 85
ventral 85
stria vascularis *60*
striosomes 84
subacute combined degeneration of cord *70*, 71
subarachnoid haemorrhage 43
subarachnoid space *10*, 40
subcortical visual areas 56–7
subdural space *10*
subiculum 98
substance P (SP) 51, 53, 111
substantia gelatinosa *32*, *50*
substantia innominata 85
substantia nigra *34*, 35
pars compacta (SNc) 84
pars reticulata (SNr) 84
subthalamic nucleus (STN) 84
subventricular zone (SVZ) 13, 39, 103

superior colliculus *34*, 35
visual functions *56*, 57, 89
superior olivary complex (SOC) *62*, 63
super-sensitivity 27
supplementary motor area (SMA) 72, 78, 79
lesions **79**, 81
seizures arising in 81
suprachiasmatic nucleus 57, 95
sweet taste *66*, 67
Sydenham's chorea 87
swing phase, locomotion *76*, 77
sympathectomy *52*, 53
sympathetic nervous system *92*, 93
activity in anxiety *110*
synapses *14*, 15, 22
axoaxonic *14*, 15
axodendritic *14*, 15
axosomatic *14*, 15
chemical 15, 22
electrical 15, 22, 23
excitatory and inhibitory *24*, 25
synaptic cleft *14*, 15, *22*, 23
synaptic integration *24*, 25
synaptic transmission 22–3
synaptic vesicle 22, 23
syringomyelia 51, *70*, 71

taste 66–7
receptors *66*, 67
transduction *66*, 67
τ protein 113
tectorial membrane (TM) *60*, 61
tectospinal tract (TeST) *32*, 33, 73, *76*, 77
temazepam 97
temperature perception, testing 105
temporal coding 45
temporal cortex 68
temporal lobe *10*, 11
epilepsy 67, 99, *114*, 115
function assessment 105
temporal summation *24*, 25
tendon reflexes 75, 105
tenth cranial nerve *see* vagus nerve
thalamus *10*, 11
lateral geniculate nucleus (LGN) 56, 57, 58–9
lesions *70*, 71
medial geniculate nucleus (MGN) *62*, 63
nociceptive pathways *50*, 51
olfactory projections 67
ventroanterior–ventrolateral nuclei (VA–VL) 84
ventroposterior (VP) nucleus *48*, 49
vestibular pathways *64*
thermal thresholds 107
thermoreceptors 51
thermoregulation 95
third cranial nerve *see* oculomotor nerve
third ventricle *40*
thirst 95
thoracic nerves *10*, 11
tight junctions 16, 41
tongue *66*, 67
tonotopic organization *62*, 63
touch
assessment *104*, 105
receptors *48*, 49
tractus solitarius *34*, 35
transcortical reflexes 81

transcutaneous electrical nerve stimulation (TENS) *52*, 53
transducin 46
transient ischaemic attacks 43
transmembrane pore 19
transverse myelitis *70*, 71
transverse tubules (T-tubules) 28, 30–1
tremor
palatal 83
in Parkinson's disease 86
triads *28*, 29, 31
tricyclic antidepressants 109, 110
trigeminal nerve (fifth cranial nerve) *36*, 37
assessment *104*, 105
trigeminal neuralgia 53
trigeminal sensory system *48*, 49
trinucleotide (triplet) repeat disorders 118, 119
trk receptors *100*, 101
trochlear nerve (IV) 36
assessment *104*, 105
tropomyosin *28*, 29, 30, 31
troponin *28*, 29, 30, 31
T-tubules 28, 30–1
twelfth cranial nerve *see* hypoglossal nerve
tympanic membrane *60*, 61

ulnar nerve entrapment 71
upper motorneurone (UMN) lesions 73, *90*, 91
up-regulation, receptor 27
utricle *64*, 65

vagus (tenth) nerve *36*, 37
assessment *104*, 105
valproate, sodium 115
vasculitides 117
vasopressin (antidiuretic hormone) 94
venous drainage, brain 43
ventral (anterior) root *10*, 11, 32
ventral spinocerebellar tract (VSCT) *76*, 77
ventral tegmental area 85
ventromedial motor system *76*, 77
ventroposterior (VP) nucleus of thalamus *48*, 49
verbal fluency 104
vertebrae *10*, 11
vertebral arteries *42*, 43
vertebral column *10*, 11
vertigo, benign positional 65
vesicles, synaptic 22, 23
vestibular nuclei *34*, 35, *64*, 65, 89
vestibular reflexes 65
vestibular system 64–5
central 65
peripheral disorders 65
vestibular transduction *64*, 65
vestibulocochlear nerve (eighth cranial nerve) *36*, 37, 63
assessment *104*, 105
vestibulo-ocular reflex 65, *102*, 103
vestibulospinal tract (VeST) *64*, *76*, 77, **121**
in motor control *72*, 73
spinal cord *32*, 33
vibration perception threshold (VPT) testing *104*, 105
vigabatrin 115
vision, blurred 89
visual acuity 55
visual cortex 58–9
extrastriate (association) areas 56, *58*, 59, 69, 89

visual cortex (*cont.*)
    primary (V1, Brodmann's area 17)   56, 57,
        58–9, 89
visual-evoked potentials (VEPs)
        107
visual field defects   56–7
visual pathways   56–7
    lesions   56–7
visual system   54–9

phototransduction   *46*, 47
    plasticity in developing   102–3
visuospatial function   105
vitamin B$_{12}$ deficiency   71

Wallenberg's lateral medullary syndrome
        43
Wallerian degeneration   *100*, 101
water balance   95

weakness   90–1
    pyramidal distribution   73, 77
Wernicke's area   *42*, *62*, 63
white matter   *10*, 11
Wilson's disease   87

XYW retinal ganglion cells   55

zopiclone   97